FIT AGAIN

FIT AGAIN

90 Days to Lifetime Fitness for the Over-35 Male

Royce Flippin

Exercise Photographs by Kevin Kuenster

A Birch Lane Press Book
Published by Carol Publishing Group

A Birch Lane Press Book
Published by Carol Publishing Group
Birch Lane Press is a registered trademark of Carol
Communications, Inc.

Editorial Offices: 600 Madison Avenue,
New York, N.Y. 10022
Sales and Distribution Offices: 120 Enterprise Avenue,
Secaucus, N.J. 07094
In Canada: Canadian Manda Group, One Atlantic
Avenue, Suite 105, Toronto, Ontario M6K 3E7

Queries regarding rights and permissions should be
addressed to Carol Publishing Group,
600 Madison Avenue, New York, N.Y. 10022.

Carol Publishing Group books are available at special
discounts for bulk purchases, sales promotion, fund-
raising, or educational purposes. Special editions can
be created to specifications. For details, contact:
Special Sales Department, Carol Publishing Group,
120 Enterprise Avenue, Secaucus, N.J. 07094.

Manufactured in the United States of America

10 9 8 7 6 5 4 3 2 1

Library of Congress Cataloging-in-Publication Data

Flippin, Royce.
    Fit again : 90 days to lifetime fitness for the over-35
male / Royce Flippin.
        p.   cm.
    "A Birch Lane Press book."
    ISBN 1-55972-321-1
    1. Physical fitness for men. 2. Exercise for men.
I. Title.
GV482.5.F55   1995
613.7'0449—dc20   95-19226
                                            CIP

CONTENTS

ACKNOWLEDGMENTS

I'd like to thank my family and friends, and especially my parents, for their support of this book project. I'd also like specifically to thank the following people for contributing their knowledge of health and fitness: Wayne Westcott, Jane Katz, Bob Barnett, Jim Bolster, Tom Brunick, Casey Meyers, John Duncan, Miram Nelson, John Blievernicht, Marjorie Koutsandreas, Barbara Wiegand, David Imrie, Daniel Kosich, Mary Pullig Schatz, Jonathan Smith, James Rippe, and Murray Hamlet.

Finally, thanks to Rebecca Norris, John Reiners, and Jim Burke for their help—and many thanks, of course, to my editor Jim Ellison, without whom this book would not have happened.

PREFACE

What if you had a beautiful car that had gotten dusty and out of tune with neglect—but that you could have up and running again with just a few weeks of attention?

If this were true, you would have already done it, right? Well, here's some news for you: *Your muscles are just like that prize car.*

No matter how long it's been since you did any regular exercise, your muscles (including your heart) are still just as responsive to it today as they were when you were 20. Start training them on a regular basis, and you'll see gains in both strength and endurance, beginning within two or three weeks. Stick with it for three months, and your body will literally transform itself before your eyes.

This is true *no matter what age you are.* In a recent study at Tufts University, men and women in their eighties more than *doubled* their strength after a twelve-week weight-lifting program, improving their agility and mobility remarkably in the process.

The same is true where your aerobic endurance is concerned. Doctors find that bedridden patients, who are as out of shape as anyone can be, can quickly double or even triple their aerobic capacity to utilize oxygen with a couple of months of regular, light exercise. To put this in perspective: If you're totally out of shape, you'll show much more *relative* improvement in your aerobic ability after three months of a regular exercise program than will an athlete in heavy training (who would be happy with a 5 or 10 percent improvement).

At the same time, you'll also be increasing your life span. In April 1995, some startling news appeared on the front page of the *New York Times:* After following 17,000 male Harvard graduates for almost three decades, researchers had identified the biggest single factor in extending life. The magic prescription—a half-hour a day of vigorous exercise. That exercise could include walking, cycling, lap swimming, jogging, or hard tennis, as long it was done on a daily or near-daily basis. The men in the study who followed this prescription and burned 1,500 calories a week or more by exercising had a 25 percent lower death rate from 1962 through 1988 than those in the study who expended *less* than 1,500 per week. The Harvard analysis concluded that this difference was due mainly to a reduced rate of heart attacks and cardiovascular disease, since regular exercise improves cholesterol levels and also enhances general circulation.

So there it is, in black and white. If you really want to maximize your health, and share as many years as you can with your family and friends, you'll need to start working out.

Yeah, you say, but a half-hour every day? Who has the time?

The answer is, *you* do—if you know where to look for it. And that's what this book is all about. It will help you over-35 males map out a weekly exercise plan and show you how to include "no-sweat" workouts that can fit around your work schedule.

As a first step toward this goal, you'll need to start rethinking your notions about what "exercise" is. Many men played sports when they were younger, and they tend to compare their present-day fitness to that idyllic time. But the fact is, athletic fitness is not the same as being fit for life. Athletic training is designed to help you excel in a specific competitive activity—which brings health benefits, but also risks. Exercising for health, on the other hand, is strictly noncompetitive—and can even be fun! Done right, it should give you all the positive benefits you're looking for without any risk of getting injured, or overtired, or burned out mentally.

Some careful studies have shown, for example, that if you walk fifteen miles each week at a steady pace—something almost anyone reading this book can do with little trouble—you will improve your cholesterol profile and significantly reduce your body fat.

If this sounds too easy, that's probably because of the American myth that "winning is everything." If you're not a highly trained athlete, this thinking goes, you're not *really* exercising—so why bother at all? This notion is completely untrue, but it's been reinforced by television, which has a parallel myth: Unless someone is doing something that *looks* unusual, like jogging along a trail or working out at a health club, viewers won't think they're watching *real* exercise. (After all, everyone walks, right?)

In fact *all* movement is "real" exercise, and the normal activities you're involved in already can be easily shaped into a workable, life-extending exercise program. The *Fit Again* program puts you—the over-35 male concerned about your present state of fitness—in the driver's seat, by telling you exactly how and why exercise is good for you, and how much you need to stay in top-notch health.

Thirty-five years old may seem too young to start worrying about what you eat or how much you exercise. But autopsies of soldiers killed in combat have shown that fatty streaks in the arteries (an early sign of heart disease) can show up when men are in their mid-thirties, or even younger.

Your thirties are also the time when shifts in body composition—to more body fat and less muscle mass—first start to appear. "No one is sure how much of this is a natural consequence of getting older, and how much is due to a decline in physical activity," says Dr. Roger Fielding, a researcher at the Tufts University Center for Nutrition and Aging. "We've found that men in their twenties are habitually very active, even when they say they don't exercise. But there's a big drop in habitual activity in the ten-year span from age 25 to age 35."

According to Fielding, 35 is also when men first begin to show noticeable declines in aerobic functioning and lean muscle mass—changes that can eventually lead to cardiovascular disease, diabetes, and even cancer. "The real declines don't occur until later decades—but the thirties is where they start," he says. "It's really the best time to initiate an exercise program, so you can prevent the gradual deterioration from ever getting started."

It's natural to lose a little bit of your edge in middle age. But there's one big shift that *doesn't* have to happen. It starts when layers of fat appear on your abdomen, back, and upper arms. At the same time, you start tiring more quickly at sports or when you're out walking, and maybe your back starts to act up a little—until gradually you find yourself sitting around watching television more and more, at times when you used to be up and moving!

The problem is simple. By not being active enough, you've lost your *aerobic muscle power.* Aerobic muscle power is the long-term endurance of the large muscles in your legs, hips, buttocks, and trunk. This is the power that carries you everywhere, whether you're walking, running, swimming, skiing, playing tennis, or buying groceries. The only time you're not working aerobically is when you're asleep, or sitting at a desk, in a car, or in an armchair—which for most Americans is too much of the time.

When your large muscle groups are exercised regularly, they're stimulated to grow more tiny oxygen conversion units called *mitochondria.* Mitochondria are cells where oxygen and sugar are turned into the energy that muscles burn every time they contract. These cells are microscopic powerhouses. The bigger and more numerous they become, the fitter your muscles will be.

The proportion of mitochondria in your own muscles changes depending on how much exercise they've been getting. If you're like most men, your level of physical activity has slowly trailed off as the responsibilities of adulthood grew. As you neglect your muscles, your mitochondria gradually diminish in size and number, and your muscles become much less effective at turning oxygen into energy.

It's not a loss you notice until you find yourself breathless during a game of basketball, or after you climb a long flight of stairs—and suddenly you think, boy, am I out of shape! It doesn't take long to get your aerobic power back, though. If you start exercising your muscles daily, following the "Harvard prescription" of a half-hour per day, your muscles will immediately start upgrading their mitochondria supply, along with key enzymes that help your muscles burn fats and carbohydrates more effectively. And as your muscles upgrade their oxygen-burning capacity, other changes happen too:

- More capillaries (tiny blood vessels that feed your muscle fibers) sprout up, increasing by up to 50 percent with heavy training.

- Your heart muscle will also grow stronger and pump more blood with each contraction.
- Your blood plasma will become slightly more diluted, flowing more easily through your capillaries (which also lessens the chance of dangerous blood clots).
- Most important of all, your levels of HDL cholesterol will rise. HDL is the "good" cholesterol, working as a protective scavenger in your arteries to prevent plaque from blocking blood flow to your heart. Your ratio of HDL cholesterol to total cholesterol is the *single best predictor* of whether or not you'll have a heart attack. (To learn more about cholesterol ratio, turn to Week Thirteen.)

It's important to realize that these beneficial changes happen *whether or not you lose any weight.* If you exercise on a regular basis, your body will undergo a dynamic transformation in just a few weeks.

In fact, the first three months of any new exercise program are where your biggest improvements will occur. After 90 days, you can expect to have improved your aerobic power by as much as a third. You'll still continue to make steady gains throughout your first year of exercise (before levelling off somewhat), but about *half* of your long-term aerobic improvement will happen in the first 90 days of training.

What better investment could you make over the next three months? They'll be months well-spent for other reasons, too. As you raise your aerobic fitness, you'll also cut your risk of a heart attack in half, you'll significantly lower your risk of diabetes and colon cancer, you'll have a much easier time reducing body fat, and you'll raise your life expectancy! If you decide to add some strength training to your program, you'll also gain muscle mass and speed the fat-reducing process.

This probably sounds good to you, but you might not be sure what to do next. Relax, because you're about to find out. Just turn the page—and let the Fit Again 90-Day Program help you start getting the exercise you (and your muscles) need.

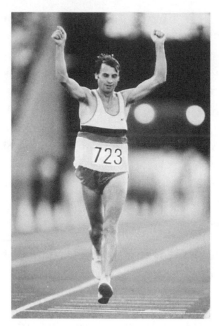

Your muscles are primed for exercise at any age. In fact, scientists now believe that *lack of physical activity* is the main reason people lose endurance and gain fat as they get older. One example of this new thinking is Carlos Lopes, the Portuguese distance runner who won a smashing victory in the 1984 Olympic marathon in Los Angeles at age 37—after many "experts" said he was ten years over the hill. *Duomo, Paul J. Sutton (© 1984)*

THE FIT AGAIN 90-DAY PROGRAM

Okay—ready to aerobicize? The Fit Again program is a progressive plan, designed to bring you gradually into the mainstream of aerobic exercise without overstressing your body. It advises choosing one primary aerobic activity (like walking, cycling, or swimming) and beginning with very short doses of this exercise (15 to 30 minutes). You'll increase the length of these aerobic workouts gradually, until by Week Six you'll have built up to three and half hours a week—the amount of exercise needed for maximum health.

The Fit Again 90-Day Program is intended as a guideline, to give you a starting point that you can work from. If the workouts seem too demanding, simply scale them down to a more comfortable length. The important thing is to get out and moving.

The first 90 days of a new exercise program are always the trickiest, for several reasons:

■ First, you'll be exploring new territory, trying to find the activities, equipment, and routine that work best for you.

■ Second, this period is the time when you're most vulnerable to injury, since your bones and tendons haven't had time to adjust fully to the daily impact of exercise. As they do, you'll need to build up your training time gradually. (For more advice on avoiding injury, see Week Three.)

■ A third reason is that one out of every two new exercisers will quit within six months and go back to a sedentary life-style—usually because of specific problems, like poorly fitted shoes, bad time management, or picking the wrong aerobic activity.

The best way to stick with your program is to begin slowly and keep your exercise routine as enjoyable and hassle-free as you can. This book will guide you through these all-important first three months and give you the tools and knowledge to shape your own exercise program in the months and years that follow.

What You Can Expect

The Fit Again plan does *not* recommend:

■ restricting the amount of calories you eat each day,
■ aiming for a specific weight loss goal,
■ trying for a "target heart rate" during exercise,
■ doing any high-impact exercise, like running, until after you've completed this 90-day startup period.

The Fit Again program *does* recommend:

■ working to build muscle mass, which will help to reduce body fat,
■ committing yourself to five aerobic workouts a week, done at a moderate, enjoyable pace,
■ doing one long aerobic session each week,
■ taking your resting heart rate once a day, as a gauge of your fitness (simply count the heartbeats in 30 seconds and multiply by 2),

- cutting down on the percentage of fat in your diet, especially saturated fats and hydrogenated fats.

The plan is divided into three phases:

Weeks one through four make up the initiation phase, when your body and muscles will still be adapting to your new aerobic life-style. Workouts build slowly in length during this phase and call for an easy-to-moderate pace. You may feel slightly more tired than usual in these first weeks, as your body adjusts to the new stress of daily exercise.

Weeks five through eight are the build-up phase, when you'll see the most dramatic changes in your body, especially in your muscle size and tone. You'll reach your final goal of three-and-a-half hours of aerobic training per week during this phase. Pace should be moderate throughout these middle weeks.

Weeks nine through thirteen represent consolidation. This third phase will feature continued steady improvement in your aerobic endurance. If you choose to follow the strength training segment of the program, you'll also continue to show increases in muscle size. This phase continues the aerobic training load of the previous months, but emphasizes more brisk walking.

If you stick to your plan, you'll see signs of enhanced fitness as early as the second or third week. As you progress from week to week, look for these signs of improvement:

- your resting heart rate will go *down,*
- your ability to do exercise without getting short of breath will go *up,*
- your muscle tone and energy level will improve,
- your fat will start to melt away!

Besides stressing aerobic exercise, the Fit Again program will also help you increase your strength and range of motion in your muscles and joints. Each week, special "Workout Adviser" and "Body Maintenance Manual" sections will introduce you to the basic techniques of strength training, stretching, and "variable paced" workouts like interval training. You'll also find advice on strengthening your back muscles and the muscles you use in balancing, as well as tips on buying a pair of exercise shoes, scheduling your workouts, healtly eating, how to handle the heat and the cold, and much more.

This training schedule is laid out one week at a time in a calendar format, so you can record your exercise sessions right in this book. At the end of 90 days, you'll have a convenient diary of your progress!

The training calendar has space for you to describe your workout for the day and also to record any comments about how you felt physically, what the day was like, and so on. You'll also see a space for you to write down your resting heart rate (Resting HR) each day. This is the number of times your heart beats in a minute, as you sit relaxed in a chair or lie in bed.

Finally, you'll also see a checklist with each week's training schedule. This checklist isn't meant to be actually marked off—it's there as a reminder of the most basic elements of the Fit Again philosophy.

The first item on the checklist asks whether you did *some* aerobic activity at least five times during the week. Even if you can't work out as much as the Fit Again plan calls for, you should aim for a minimum exercise session each day. At the start of the program, this minimum is 15 minutes. Over the next six weeks it increases to at least 30 minutes of aerobic exercise per day (except on rest days).

The second item asks, "Did I get in one long aerobic workout?" The Fit Again plan recommends one weekly aerobic session that's a little longer than the others—one that lasts an hour, or more once you've built up to your full training load. Steadily walking, cycling, or swimming for an hour-plus will improve your blood flow and burn fat in a way that shorter workouts won't. There's also a psychological benefit from pushing yourself a little farther than you usually go.

The last item on the checklist is, "Did I make healthy choices in what I did and ate?" Once you start exercising regularly, you'll find that you're not as quick to deprive yourself of sleep, or put toxins into your body, including cigarettes and alcohol. This item is a reminder to treat your body well, and especially to avoid eating harmful fats whenever possible (for details on a healthy eating plan, see Week Four).

Before You Start

Your first stop in your new aerobic program should be a visit to your regular doctor, where you can share your exercise plans and get a thorough checkup, including a blood pressure exam and a cardiovascular evaluation. The American Medical Association advises *everyone* over age 35 to get a complete medical checkup before starting a new exercise program. This is doubly important if you've smoked in the past, are overweight, or have a family history of heart disease.

Your doctor will probably be pleased by your decision to exercise regularly. The chief caution you're likely to get is, don't try to do too much too fast—which is also the philosophy of the Fit Again program.

Taking the First Step

Before you get underway for real, you should read Week One, which discusses how to select workout shoes and gives some technical tips on fitness walking. But if you like, you can get a jump on your new program right now. Simply put this book down, change into a comfortable pair of shoes, and go for a casual 15-minute walk, wherever you happen to be—in your yard, down the street, to the neighborhood park and back. It doesn't matter, as long as your walking route is smooth and relatively traffic-free.

Have a nice walk! When you get back you'll have completed the first day of the Fit Again 90-Day Program . . . and your muscles will already be starting their transformation.

THE FIT AGAIN 90-DAY PLAN, AT A GLANCE

MONTH 1 (WEEKS 1–4)

Aerobic Workouts (minutes)	Time (Calories)	Strength Workouts
1. 15 / 15 / 20 / 20 / 30	1:40 (600–800)	none
2. 20 / 20 / 25 / 25 / 40	2:10 (780–1040)	none
3. 20 / 20 / 30 / 30 / 45	2:25 (870–1160)	2 (1–2 sets)
4. 25 / 25 / 35 / 35 / 45	2:45 (990–1320)	2 (1–2 sets)

MONTH 2 (WEEKS 5–8)

Aerobic Workouts (minutes)	Time (Calories)	Strength Workouts
5. 30 / 30 / 45 / 45 / 45	3:15 (1170–1560)	2 (1–2 sets)
6. 30 / 30 / 45 / 45 / 60	3:30 (1260–1680)	2 (1–2 sets)
7. 30 / 30 / 45 / 45 / 60	3:30 (1260–1680)	2 (1–2 sets)
8. 30 / 30 / 45 / 45 / 60	3:30 (1260–1680)	2+(1–2 sets)

MONTH 3 (WEEKS 9–13)

Aerobic Workouts (minutes)	Time (Calories)	Strength Workouts
9. 30 / 30 / 45 / 45 / 60+	3:30+ (1260–1680+)	2+(1–2 sets)
10. 30 / 30 / 45 / 45 / 60+	3:30+ (1260–1680+)	2+(1–2 sets)
11. 30 / 30 / 45 / 45 / 60+	3:30+ (1260–1680+)	2+(1–2 sets)
12. 30 / 30 / 45 / 45 / 60+	3:30+ (1260–1680+)	2+(1–2 sets)
13. 30 / 30 / 45 / 45 / 60+	3:30+ (1260–1680+)	2+(1–2 sets)

FIT AGAIN

WEEK ONE

(DAYS 1–7)

TWO 15–MINUTE WORKOUTS

TWO 20–MINUTE WORKOUTS

ONE 30–MINUTE WORKOUT

(NO STRENGTH WORKOUTS)

Total aerobic time: 1:40 (100 minutes)

Total calories burned: 600 calories if you weigh 165 lbs.; 700 calories, 190 lbs.; 800 calories, 220 lbs.

WEEKLY CHECKLIST

☐ Did I do at least 15 minutes of aerobic activity five times this week?

☐ Did I get in one long aerobic workout?

☐ Did I make healthy choices in what I did and ate?

DAY	1	2	3
WORKOUT:			
COMMENTS:			
RESTING HR:			

WEEK ONE

GOAL: To begin training your muscles aerobically, with an easy schedule of 100 aerobic minutes, divided into workouts of 15, 15, 20, 20, and 30 minutes. (If you prefer, you can simply do five workouts of 20 minutes each.)

WEEKLY REPORT: Welcome to the exercising week! Week One is a very easy introduction to aerobic training—totalling just over an hour and half for the week. As you're walking or cycling, try to keep a steady but relaxed pace. When you finish, you should feel you easily could have gone twice as far if you had to. But be glad you didn't—although your muscles are eager for the work, your more fragile tendons and joint paddings have been in dry dock for a while and should be treated with care in these early weeks.

The first two weeks are also when you're likely to feel most fatigued. Remember, exercise places stress on your body—a healthy

4	5	6	7

stress, but stress all the same—and it takes a week or so for your body to adjust to the initial impact.

The biggest hurdle in this first week, though, will be psychological—you've got to get out of the habit of moving from your house to your car to your office and back again.

To see the magical powers of exercise at work, let's consider the hypothetical case history of a man called John Jones. In his early forties, John's just entering middle age. He's married, with a 12-year-old son and a 10-year-old daughter, and has a successful career as an advertising executive. He works hard, commuting from the suburbs into the city each morning (his office is in midtown, of course), and enjoys a reasonably active social life with his wife, who works part-time herself.

John is happy with the way most things are going in his life. But the condition of his body isn't one of them—because John is becoming sadly out of shape. His wife calls him "bearish," but the truth is that John is now pushing 200 pounds (more than 20 pounds heavier than he was when he graduated college), and he has a hefty spare tire of fat around his waist. He's still quick on his feet, but loses his breath a lot sooner than he used to—a fact he blames on his extra weight. He has made some half-hearted attempts to go on a diet, but his weight continues to creep upward with each passing year.

It wasn't always like this. John was an avid basketball player in high school and a gung ho intramural athlete in college. But as things stand now, the only exercise John is getting is his traditional Wednesday racketball game with a few friends and an occasional bike ride with his wife on the weekends. She now bicycles on a regular basis—and although John has always considered himself the athlete in the family, he now has to push to keep up with her on their rides together.

John's wife has noticed the changes in his body, too, and she's concerned for her own reasons: John's father suffered a heart attack in his mid-sixties, and she's determined that this won't happen to John. That's why she's been after him to get his annual checkup. He skipped last year's appointment, using business as an excuse.

This year, though, there was no avoiding the issue—which is why we find John sitting in his doctor's office bright and early on Monday morning, getting some news he'd rather not hear.

"Sit down, John," said his doctor. "Frankly, I'm unhappy with the way your tests turned out last week. Your cholesterol ratio is simply too high, and your blood pressure is slightly elevated, too. But most disturbing is your stress test. When you were walking at top speed, your heart showed signs that there may be the beginnings of a blockage in one of your coronary arteries."

John felt a chill run up his back. "What do you mean, Doc?" he said. "Am I going to have a heart attack, like my dad?"

"Not if I can help it," his doctor said. "The blockage is in a very early stage. This is the time to take action, before the problem gets any worse. If you follow this prescription to the letter, I think we should be able to stop the disease from progressing—and keep you with us for a long, long time."

The doctor scribbled on a piece of paper and handed it to John. "What is it?" John doubtfully asked. "A new sort of medication?"

"Read it," his physician answered.

John looked down and saw the doctor had written: "3 1/2 hours aerobic exercise per week; cut fats to 20% of daily food intake."

He looked up blankly. "That's it?" he said.

"That's it," the doctor replied. "But you've got to follow this advice to the letter. Begin with an hour and half the first week, and add a few minutes each week until you reach the prescribed level."

John still looked puzzled. "What kind of aerobic exercise?" he said.

"Walking, biking, swimming, the exer-cycle at the gym." The doctor shrugged. "Whatever you want, as long as you do a half-hour at a time."

"But walking isn't real exercise, is it?"

"It is if you do it every day for a half hour or more," said the doctor.

"What about the eating? How will I know what 20 percent of my daily intake means?"

The doctor glanced at his notes. "According to the nutrition diary you filled out, you take in about 2,500 calories a day, so 20 percent fats means no more than 500 calories of fat a day. There are 9 calories of fat in a gram. So that works out to 55 grams of fat a day." The doctor wrote this figure on a second piece of paper and handed it to John as well. "Most food packages will tell you exactly how much fat they contain, so you can count the grams as you go."

John sat clutching the two pieces of paper as if they were tickets to an amusement park ride he wasn't sure he wanted to take. "It's that easy?" he said finally.

His doctor stood up and opened the office door as John rose to leave. "I didn't say it would be easy," the physician said. "Just essential. I'll see you again in a few weeks."

John walked down the hallway still holding the two slips of paper in his free hand. He felt strangely relieved, as if a new future was waiting up ahead. He just wasn't clear yet on exactly how he was going to get there.

Workout Adviser: Evaluating Your Fitness

As part of your checkup, your doctor might choose to give you an exercise stress test, like the one given to our mythical John Jones. A stress test usually involves 10 or 15 minutes of pedalling on a stationary bike or walking on a treadmill, while the tester raises the level of effort every few minutes. Eventually the exerciser reaches the point of exhaustion, usually when his heart rate reaches about 85 percent of maximum.

By recording the subject's heart rate on an electrocardiograph before and during the exercise, a doctor can often spot abnormal heartbeats that signal some kind of artery blockage—the hallmark of heart disease.

About 80 percent of advanced cases of heart disease are discovered by stress tests. If your stress test is negative, you most likely don't have any serious blockages—but it's *not* a guarantee that you're free of heart disease.

Stress tests will also uncover exercise-related high blood pressure and will provide a good estimate of your aerobic capacity (or VO_2 max—the maximum amount of oxygen your body can utilize at one time). This figure is an indication of how fit you are.

If you don't get a full-fledged stress test, you can still evaluate your own aerobic fitness with the following One-Mile Walking Test, developed by Dr. James Rippe of Tufts University and his colleagues. You can repeat this test whenever you want to, to check your improvement from week to week. Here's how:

1. Rest completely the day before taking this test. On the day of the test, don't eat, smoke, or drink coffee or tea for at least two hours before the test.

2. Find a wristwatch that indicates seconds, and practice taking your pulse rate with it. Placing your fingertips on the base of your wrist, on the side nearest your thumb, count the number of heartbeats in 30 seconds, and multiply by 2.

3. Find a quarter-mile track, or a smooth, flat path that has one mile marked off on it. (Use a car odometer to measure a mile on the road, if you have to.)

4. Walk slowly for 10 minutes or so (until you're perspiring slightly) to get your blood flowing to your muscles.

5. Walk one mile at a steady pace, and record your time in minutes and seconds. Then immediately take your pulse rate.

6. Using your time and your pulse rate, locate your fitness on the chart below.

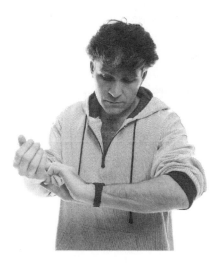

How hard your heart beats after a moderate walk is a sign of how fit you are. As you get in better shape, your heart rate will go down, both at rest and when you're exercising.

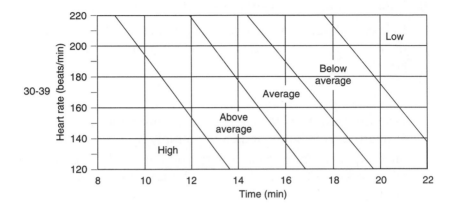

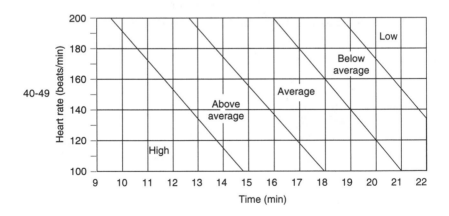

Select the fitness chart that matches your age. *Reprinted by permission of Dr. James Rippe*

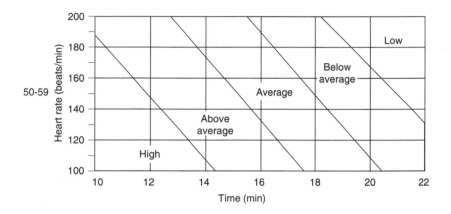

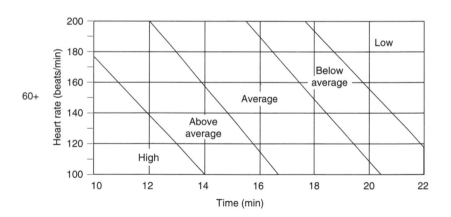

Body Maintenance Manual: Buying Exercise Shoes

If you plan to be spending several hours a week walking, playing tennis, or doing any other weight-bearing exercise, it's important to pick out a pair of workout shoes that fit your feet exactly and that provide the type of support and push-off best suited to the way your body is constructed. "I've seen more people quit exercising because they were wearing the wrong shoe than for any other reason," says Tom Brunick, director of the Athlete's Foot Test Wear Center at North Central College in Naperville, Illinois.

Brunick evaluates the newest athletic shoes each year. It's a job that gets bigger all the time: Today there are more brands and varieties of sports shoes on the market than ever before. When you walk into a shoe store that has hundreds of different sneakers for sale, be prepared to spend a little time narrowing down the field.

A good starting point is to shop for shoes only in an established athletic shoe store, such as the Athlete's Foot, Herman's, and Foot Locker chains. Look for attentive salesmen who are familiar with their stock and will take the time to measure your feet and discuss your exercise plans.

"Ignore the big wall of shoes," says Brunick. "Go right to a salesperson and explain what you're looking for. And be sure they measure your feet—not just the length of your foot, but also your foot's width, and the length of your arch. If they don't—walk on out of there!"

Once you feel secure that you've found the right store, you can use the following tips to zero in on that perfect pair of shoes, the ones that will make you feel like you could walk forever:

- Pay no attention to the hype about "amazing new breakthroughs." Today's shoes are well-constructed, with many ingenious features, but most of these features—like air pockets and stability plugs in the heel, and lightweight shock-absorbent midsoles—have been around for years. The latest "new" products from Adidas, Nike, New Balance, and the other big companies tend to be subtle variations on the previous year's model.

APPROPRIATE SHOE CATEGORIES FOR VARIOUS ACTIVITIES:

Walking: walking shoe, light hiking shoe, or light running shoe

Cycling: cycling shoe, walking shoe with leather upper, or light running or cross-training shoe with leather upper

Stationary bike: walking shoe, light running shoe, or cross-training shoe

Aerobic dance: aerobics shoe

Running: running shoe

Weight lifting: walking shoe, running shoe, cross-training shoe

Basketball, tennis, racketball: court shoe

- Expect to spend between $50 and $80 for a well-made athletic shoe. If you spend less, you're probably getting an inferior product. You can also spend more—well over $100 in the case of some running shoes—but these top-end models usually offer more support and protection than the average person needs.

- Buy a shoe designed specifically for your primary form of exercise. Athletic shoes are specialized, for good reason. Walking and running shoes are designed to do just that—move forward in a straight line. Tennis and basketball sneakers, on the other hand, will give you great support in stop-and-go, side-to-side action, but they don't have the right type of cushioning *or* enough flexibility to take you through 30 minutes of walking or running. The same goes for cross-training shoes.

- A good fit is critical. Insist on actually walking around the store to test any new pair of shoes you try on. Your shoe should fit snugly in the heel, to prevent your feet from pulling out as you walk or run. The toe box should be roomy enough for you to wiggle your toes slightly, and there should be at least a quarter-inch between your longest toe and the front of the shoe. Also, be careful that the arch support is placed appropriately for your foot, since arches differ widely from one brand to another. If you have especially wide or narrow feet, look for brands that come in variable widths, like New Balance and Rockport.

- Buy a shoe appropriate to your weight. The heavier you are, the more support you'll need. Lighter men can get by with a lighter, more flexible shoe.

- Check the flexibility of the shoes you're considering. Any walking or running shoe *must* have sufficient flexibility through the ball of the foot, otherwise you can strain the tendons on the bottom of your foot. Pick up each shoe you examine, turn it over, and try bending it in your hands: It should bend fairly easily in the forefoot. If it takes an effort to bend, look for a more flexible model. (If the shoe bends all the way down to the heel, then it's *too* flexible.)

- Finally, you need a shoe that's constructed for the way your feet move as they land and push off from the ground. Everyone's feet roll inward (pronate) as they step and push off, but the degree of pronation varies quite a bit from person to person. The more you pronate, the more lateral stability and support you'll need from a shoe and the straighter the "last" should be. If you don't pronate very much, you'll do better in a more flexible, less reinforced shoe with a slightly curved "last" that will let you maximize your natural foot-roll.

  One way to see how much you pronate is to look at an old pair of sneakers: If they're worn down so that both shoes slant inward, you're a heavy pronator. If your worn shoes slope down toward the outer heel, you don't pronate very much.

- Once you find a model that works for you, stick with it. However, you should replace your walking shoes with a fresh pair at least every 700 miles (once a year or so, if you're walking consistently), or sooner if they look excessively worn down on the bottom of the heel, or if the heel counter or the insole is visibly compressed. If you're a runner, your shoes should be replaced more often—about every 500 miles.

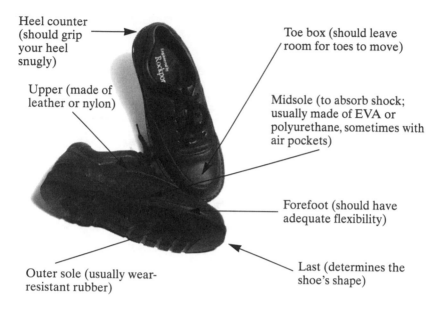

Heel counter (should grip your heel snugly)

Upper (made of leather or nylon)

Toe box (should leave room for toes to move)

Midsole (to absorb shock; usually made of EVA or polyurethane, sometimes with air pockets)

Forefoot (should have adequate flexibility)

Outer sole (usually wear-resistant rubber)

Last (determines the shoe's shape)

The Anatomy of a Workout Shoe

WEEK TWO

(D A Y S   8 – 1 4)

TWO 20-MINUTE WORKOUTS
TWO 25-MINUTE WORKOUTS
ONE 40-MINUTE WORKOUT
(NO STRENGTH WORKOUTS)

Total aerobic time: 2:10 (130 minutes)

Total calories burned: 780 calories if you weigh 165 lbs.; 910 calories, 190 lbs.; 1040 calories, 220 lbs.

WEEKLY CHECKLIST

☐ Did I do at least 20 minutes of aerobic activity five times this week?

☐ Did I get in one long aerobic workout?

☐ Did I make healthy choices in what I did and ate?

DAY	8	9	10
WORKOUT:			
COMMENTS:			
RESTING HR:			

WEEK TWO

GOAL: To continue your body's adjustment to daily aerobic exercise, by gradually increasing your aerobic "dose."

WEEKLY REPORT: Congratulations! You're now in the second week of a daily exercise program—which is more than most over-35 American men can say. You're probably slightly fatigued this week and may find yourself sleeping more soundly than usual. Remember, anytime your body is faced with the impact of a new stress, there's a physical letdown at first.

This week continues your adjustment phase, adding five or ten minutes onto each workout. Maintain an easy-to-moderate pace all week. Concentrate on relaxing and enjoying your exercise time.

This is exactly what John Jones has been trying to do. In fact, John's first two weeks went very smoothly. Two days during the week he took a slightly earlier train than usual and took a 15-minute detour on the way to his office, walking through a nearby park. He got in his Wednesday lunchtime racketball as well and then capped the week with a 30-minute bike ride on Saturday, with his wife. By the time he hit Sunday of Week 1, he felt more wiped out

11	12	13	14

than he thought he would. But he was sleeping well at night and looking forward to feeling more fit as each day went by.

John's second week was basically a replay of the first. He was helped by good weather, a fairly light workload, and the fact that his weekly racketball had kept him fit enough that he was already starting to rebound from "exercise shock." He felt more energetic and calmer by the end of Week 2.

Workout Adviser: The Fit Again Weekly Planner

Three and a half hours a week is exactly 30 minutes a day, and so it's very tempting to simply schedule a daily half-hour walk. If this approach works best for you, then go with it. However, the Fit Again program recommends *five exercise days*, and *two rest days* per week. Studies have shown that injury rates go up when people exercise six or seven days a week, compared to five. A couple of rest days each week provides some extra recovery time and adds flexibility to your exercise schedule.

This program begins with very short workouts. In the first week, you'll do 15- to 30-minute sessions of easy aerobic exercise. The workouts get progressively longer each week, and by the middle of the second month you'll be getting your full quota of aerobic exercise.

Each of the thirteen weeks follows this design:

- two "short" aerobic workouts per week,
- two "medium" aerobic workouts per week,
- one "long" aerobic workout per week,
- two weight-lifting sessions per week (starting in Week 3),
- two rest days per week.

This arrangement has a number of advantages. Short workouts let you exploit spare moments that suddenly arise during the day. And doing one longer workout each week (usually on the weekend) lets you make up for lost exercise time earlier in the week and also gives you some added physical benefits by pushing your muscles a little farther than they usually go.

Ultimately, it's up to you to schedule your exercise sessions. Start by realizing that anytime you need to walk somewhere, it's an opportunity for aerobic exercise. Then begin making your own opportunities. It may mean stealing a half-hour walk during your lunch hour or skipping a ride home from the train station at night.

You can use the Fit Again weekly calendar to help you plan your sessions and keep track of your progress—but *only you* can stick to your exercise plan. If you do, your body will thrive on it.

Body Maintenance Manual: Walking Tips

Developing a regular exercise schedule is a crucial part of the Fit Again 90-Day Program. The first step is to choose your primary aerobic exercise—the one exercise you'll do most days when you work out.

Whatever activity you choose, it has be something you can do easily, nearly every day. Why? Because it takes *repeated* exercise to condition your muscles. Exercising once every few weeks makes no more sense than watering a parched lawn once a month in the hot summer. Your muscles are like that lawn—ready and waiting to be "watered." All *you* need to do is give them regular dousings of exercise.

This exercise *doesn't* have to be strenuous. You can get excellent results by briskly walking, cycling, swimming laps, jogging, or even doing vigorous yard work on a regular basis.

There's a catch, though: While any sustained aerobic activity is good for your heart, the long-term muscular benefits of exercise occur *only* in the muscles used in that activity. This means there's very little carry-over effect from one sport to another. If you become a superfit walker, it will have only a slight effect on your swimming stamina, which depends mostly on the fitness of your arm muscles.

For this reason, the Fit Again program suggests choosing one primary aerobic activity, which can be supplemented by other types of exercise for variety.

Aerobic Rule #1: If you're out of breath, you're exercising too hard.

Aerobic Rule #2: A longer, easier workout is more effective than a short, hard one.

Choosing an Aerobic Activity

The start of a new exercise program is a good time to experiment with various exercise modes, to see what works best for you. It is important to pick an aerobic activity that you *look forward to.* If you like pedaling an exercise bike while you watch the evening news, that's great. But while a gleaming new machine may look great in your family room, most men have a hard time getting motivated to put in three and a half hours each week on stationary exercise equipment—it's just too boring.

This is why the Fit Again plan recommends choosing a real-life aerobic activity if possible, like walking, cycling, swimming (if you have access to a pool), or cross-country skiing (in the winter months)—then supplementing that activity with stationary exercise. Actively covering territory while you exercise is not only more interesting, but it also develops your postural muscles and your sense of balance in a way that stationary exercise won't.

The Fit Again plan suggests walking as your primary aerobic exercise. Thirty million people are already walking for fitness in the United States, making it the most popular aerobic sport in the country. Walking is easy and inexpensive, you can do it anywhere, it carries a very low risk of injury, and is fun and relaxing. Fitness walking also has a *proven track record* as an effective way of raising HDL cholesterol levels and reducing body fat.

(Note: The Fit Again program *doesn't* recommend running or any other high-impact sport in these first 90 days. If you want to begin a running program at the end of the three months, you and your body will be well-prepared to handle the challenge by then.)

The Walker's Guide

- Fitness walking should always be done in a comfortable, properly fitted pair of low-heeled walking shoes or light running shoes, preferably with a rubberized sole.

- Stretch very lightly before each aerobic workout—just enough to loosen up any kinks you might have. All heavy stretching should be done immediately *after* your workout, when your muscle tissues are at their warmest. (For more details on stretching exercises, see Week Five.)

- Begin each workout at a slow pace, and build up speed over the first three to four minutes—that's how long it takes for your aerobic system to fully kick in.

- Try to walk at a comfortable speed, without straining. All aerobic exercise should be done at a "conversational" pace, meaning you could carry on a conversation with a friend as you went along, if you wanted. (The exception to this is when you do interval training, discussed in Week Nine.)

  If you find yourself getting short of breath as you exercise, it's a sign that your muscles aren't getting enough oxygen—and you're starting to supplement your intake by burning anaerobic energy supplies (which are stored in the muscles themselves). Anaerobic training will help your sports performance, but it won't provide the health benefits you're after. When you "push it" during an aerobic workout, all you're really doing is tiring yourself out early and cutting short your aerobic training. You'll do better by slowing down your pace and stretching the length of your workout.

  One way to "stay aerobic" is to use the Borg scale of perceived exertion (see Appendix H). If you keep your perceived effort (how hard you feel you're working) somewhere in the range of "fairly light" to "somewhat hard" (11 to 13 on the Borg scale), you should do fine.

  Another method is to check your pulse rate. If it's over 75 percent of your *maximum* heart rate (which is roughly 220 minus your age), you should ease up on the pace of your workout. For instance, if you're 40, you have a maximum heart rate of 180 beats per minute. Three-quarters of that—or 135 beats —is your aerobic "ceiling." (See Appendix J.)

■ As you walk, concentrate on maintaining a fluid, natural stride and a smooth heel-to-toe motion with each foot. *Don't* try to make any exaggerated hip movements—the hip wiggle is for race walkers only. Keep your hips aligned and moving in a front and back direction, never side to side. Try to feel a smooth contraction in the front of your thigh and in your lower back as you push off with each leg.

■ Keep your shoulders relaxed, and hold your head upright as you walk, so you're looking forward, not down at your feet.

■ To pick up speed, *don't* lenghten your stride. Instead, bend your arms to a 90° angle at the elbow. This will shorten the "pendulum" each arm makes as it swings and let you swing your arms faster—automatically causing your stride to quicken. For full effect, bring your fist up in front of your chest with each forward arm swing, and bring it back no further than as your hip on the back swing.

With practice you can use this bent-arm technique to walk at a very fast clip. As your pace increases to 14 minutes a mile or faster, your heart beat will go up to 75 percent of your max or higher, and you'll be walking at the limits of your aerobic capacity. This is sometimes called *aerobic walking* or *power walking.*

Working at this pace will help you become a faster walker. However, *there's no evidence that very fast walking delivers any more benefits than steady, moderate walking.* When it comes to fitness walking, in other words, the important thing is to "just do it."

What about walking with handweights? In the words of Casey Meyers, walking instructor and consultant to the Institute for Aerobics Research, "Handweights have been grossly over-promoted."

Experiments have shown that handweights used with a normal walking style don't give any additional physical benefits.

The danger of handweights is that they can throw off your natural stride by lengthening it and can cause added jarring to your hips and knees as you land and push off. You can get just as good an upper body workout by using a more vigorous arm swing.

If you must use handweights use only one pound or less. As Meyers says, "If weighing yourself down really helped you to walk better, we'd all be carrying bowling balls."

You must avoid walking with ankle weights, which will completely change your stride and can cause serious injury.

Debbie Lawrence, a walking instructor and former member of the U.S. Olympic race-walking team, offers this advice.

"As you walk, imagine you have a paintbrush attached to each hip, so that it's pointing straight out to the side. Then picture yourself walking down a very narrow corridor, and try to walk so smoothly that you could paint a nice, even line along each side."

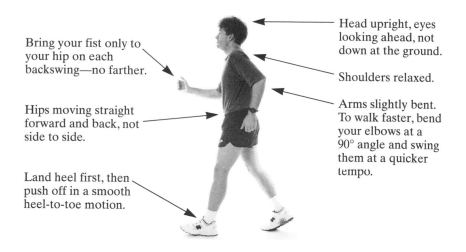

Bring your fist only to your hip on each backswing—no farther.

Hips moving straight forward and back, not side to side.

Land heel first, then push off in a smooth heel-to-toe motion.

Head upright, eyes looking ahead, not down at the ground.

Shoulders relaxed.

Arms slightly bent. To walk faster, bend your elbows at a 90° angle and swing them at a quicker tempo.

The Ideal Walking Stride

WEEK THREE

TWO 20-MINUTE WORKOUTS

TWO 30-MINUTE WORKOUTS

ONE 45-MINUTE WORKOUT

(TWO STRENGTH WORKOUTS)

Total aerobic time: 2:25 (145 minutes)

Total calories burned: 870 calories if you weigh 165 lbs.; 1015 calories, 190 lbs.; 1160 calories, 220 lbs.

WEEKLY CHECKLIST

☐ Did I do at least 20 minutes of aerobic activity five times this week?

☐ Did I get in one long aerobic workout?

☐ Did I make healthy choices in what I did and ate?

DAY	15	16	17
WORKOUT:			
COMMENTS:			
RESTING HR:			

WEEK THREE

GOAL: To continue gradually pushing your "aerobic envelope" by adding another 15 minutes of training, for a total of about two-and-a-half hours, with a long workout of 45 minutes. If you choose to, this is also an appropriate time to begin strength training twice a week.

WEEKLY REPORT: You'll be feeling much more energetic this week, as all your aerobic systems come fully on line. You should also be feeling some of the mental effects of exercise. Regular, repeated motion like walking, cycling, or swimming changes your brain in several ways: After just a few minutes it begins to stimulate the release of endorphins (technically known as endogenous opiates), which is your brain's natural way of doping itself, producing a buzz of euphoria and physical invulnerability—the fabled "exercise high."

4	5	6	7

The magnitude of this endorphin effect varies quite a bit, depending on the individual. But there's another far-reaching change that will benefit virtually anyone who exercises. Researchers have discovered that the regular, repeated motion of exercise is one of the best ways to increase brain levels of serotonin—a neurotransmitter intimately linked to feelings of well-being. Low levels of serotonin are closely connected to feelings of depression.

In this way, exercise works as a natural antidepressant medication, and it's being prescribed for that reason by many mental health practitioners. It takes about two weeks for changes in brain chemistry to affect your mood—so an emotional uplift should be kicking in right about now.

Keep the pace easy-to-moderate in all aerobic workouts this week. If you want to start a weight-lifting program, this is a good time for it. If you prefer to stick with aerobics only, that's fine, too. The Workout Adviser that follows offers some reasons why strength training will improve your health.

As for the John Jones report: He met all his aerobic goals, but it wasn't as easy as the two previous weeks. Bad weather and a busy work week forced him to go out for an extra-long bike ride with his wife on Sunday to get in his full aerobic time. He paid for his transgression when he woke up the next day with aching thigh muscles—although John's already-fit wife, to his chagrin, seemed to feel no ill effects at all.

One thing John doesn't have to worry about is what to wear: He and his wife took a trip to the local mall a few days after John's talk with his doctor and bought a lightweight sweat suit and some spanking new walking shoes. John was astonished at how light the shoes were and how well they fit—he was used to court shoes, which are heavier and less flexible than footwear designed especially for walking. To his children's amusement, he likes the shoes so much he's taken to wearing them around the house—which is actually an excellent way to break in a new pair of shoes.

Workout Adviser: Avoiding Injury

Although your muscles will adapt rapidly to new exercise, the stiffer material that connects them to your body—your tendons and joints—adjusts much more slowly. Sudden overwork, even one hard workout, can cause tendinitis or some other type of inflammation to flare up, virtually overnight. Tendinitis can occur on the bottom of your foot, in or under your knee, in the powerful muscles of your hip, or (for swimmers and tennis players) in the shoulder or elbow. The symptoms are a burning pain when you try to put weight on the affected limb and a tenderness when you touch the injured area.

Injuries can be avoided by using common sense and being careful not to overdo your exercise:

- Select walking terrain that's smooth underfoot, and wear well-fitted shoes that are appropriate to your activity.

- Begin any new form of exercise cautiously, by doing short, easy workouts, and increase your training load very gradually—no matter how strong your muscles are feeling. One good rule of thumb is to never increase the intensity and the length of your workouts at the same time.

- Be especially wary of the "super workout," when you're inspired to go farther or faster than ever before—because all too many people have injured themselves on days when they "never felt better." They found out the hard way that a single over-strenuous workout is enough to hurt you.

- You can also get hurt on days when you're below par, mentally or physically. Don't be afraid to take a rest day when your body seems to want it, especially if you're sick. Any true illness will be cured more quickly by rest than by exercise. If you have a bad cold or the flu, or if you're particularly worn out from work or lack of sleep, take a couple of days' vacation from exercise, or do a minimal (light 15-minute) workout, just to get your blood circulating a bit.

- Muscle soreness may occur when you begin exercising underused muscles, or when you do a harder-than-usual workout. Doctors have found that soreness is mostly caused by "eccentric" muscle contractions—when your muscles are moving *with* gravity as they contract. This happens, for instance, when your legs work to brake your movement—such as walking downstairs or stopping quickly on the basketball court—or when you're slowly lowering a heavy weight to the ground.

The soreness usually peaks a day or two after the offending workout and is thought to be a symptom of torn collagen (microscopic connective tissue surrounding the muscle fibers). It's also a sign that you're working your muscles too hard, or incorrectly. Rest a couple of days or do very light workouts (to help flush out the toxins), and the soreness should pass quickly.

■ If you feel a pain or muscle tightness during your workout, stop whatever you're doing *immediately*. Take all weight off the injured area, and apply ice regularly for the next 24 to 48 hours. Employ the same treatment if pain appears the day after your workout. *Don't* try to exercise again until the pain has completely subsided for at least a couple of days.

■ If the pain persists or returns, see a sports physician who's experienced in treating overuse injuries. If inflammation, such as tendinitis or bursitis, is the problem, the doctor is likely to prescribe rest and perhaps a non-steroidal anti-inflammatory drug (NSAID) such as aspirin, ibuprofen, or Indocin, which can help speed recovery.

However, a chronic pain is a clear indication of a mechanical problem—usually some kind of muscle imbalance due to weak or tight muscles, or a structural defect in the way your bones are aligned. It's important to pinpoint and treat both the pain *and* the underlying muscle weakness or tightness that's causing it. If your physician doesn't prescribe some kind of physical therapy for your injury, you should probably switch doctors.

Body Maintenance Manual: A No-frills Strength Training Program

If you're under 50, strength training probably isn't as important to your health as aerobics is. But it becomes more critical as you get older, especially as you approach 60. That's because your muscle mass will tend to decline slightly with age, starting around age 50. *Scientists now think that much of this shrinkage can be attributed to inactivity.*

Aerobic exercise alone can't reverse this process. To maintain maximum strength and size, you need to stimulate your anaerobic energy systems by "overloading" your major muscle groups two or three times a week. Overloading a muscle group is simple: You just use those muscles to lift a heavy weight 8 to 12 times in succession. The training weight should be enough to make the last repetition feel fairly difficult. If the twelfth repetition feels easy, you're not using enough weight.

Why do 8 to 12 reps instead of 20 or 25? The reason is that you want to work your target muscle to a point of fatigue within the anaerobic energy system—which is about 50 to 70 seconds for most people. Twenty or 25 repetitions would take you outside this anaerobic system (assuming you take about 6 seconds for each repetition)—which would provide a good workout, but wouldn't build any strength in the muscle.

If you're using a weight machine, one set of 8 to 12 reps is all you need. If you work out with dumbbells, you should do two sets of each exercise for maximum benefits.

Doing 8 to 12 slow, smooth repetitions takes only about a minute or so for each muscle group, and the payoff is worth the investment. Not only will your muscles get bigger, but your HDL cholesterol levels will get another boost (in addition to the increases being triggered by your aerobic program). Strength training will make you slimmer, too: Studies have shown that if you lift weights twice a week, your increased muscle mass will help hold down your fat levels *better* than aerobics alone.

If that isn't enough to sell you on weight lifting, it's also been proven to be good for your bones, keeping them strong and healthy by slowing the process of osteoporosis. And lifting weights will toughen your tendons, protecting you from injury in stop-and-go sports like softball and basketball.

Stronger leg muscles will also give you added agility and sprinting power for any sport you care to play. And like aerobics, weight lifting is extremely effective *at any age.* In a well-known study at Tufts University, men and women in their eighties and nineties more than doubled the amount they could lift, after just a dozen weeks of leg exercises similar to the ones shown here.

Getting Started

Lifting weights can seem like a complicated, time-consuming endeavor, but it's really quick and simple if you know what you're doing.

True strength training employs a variety of exercises that focus on a balanced muscular development. You'll need to do only one or two sets of each exercise—each set will take a little over a minute to complete. Strive for *slow, controlled movements* with a manageable amount of weight, getting the most out of each lift. If you train in this way, you can increase your strength rapidly on just two workouts a week.

The following 15-minute, "no-frills" strength program was recommended by Wayne Westcott, Ph.D., strength training consultant for the YMCA. It uses just four strength exercises, but it works all the important muscles used in walking, standing, and pushing and pulling with your upper body. This program can be done at home— all you need are a pair of dumbbells with adjustable weights, so you can increase the load as you get stronger. You can also do this training on weight machines, such as Nautilus, if you have access to a gym or health club.

Here are the four exercises:

Squats with dumbbells	or	Leg extensions (Nautilus)
Lunges with dumbbells	or	Leg curl (Nautilus)
Bench press with dumbbells	or	Chest press (Nautilus)
Bentover dumbbell row	or	Lat pull-down (Nautilus)

To get the most out of your strength training sessions, keep the following tips in mind:

■ Do two sets of each dumbbell exercise (if you're using weight machines, one is sufficient), repeating the movement 8 to 12 times.

■ The weight should be heavy enough to make the last repetition of each set feel fairly difficult. Westcott recommends beginning with a weight equal to about 75 percent of what you could lift in one all-out effort. If you're uncertain about where to begin, start with a 20-pound dumbbell, then add weight if this seems too light.

■ Do each repetition in a slow, controlled fashion, working through your entire range of motion. As a rule, you should take about two seconds to lift a weight and four seconds to lower it. You should try to use as full a movement as possible as you do: This is more difficult, but much more productive in terms of stimulating and strengthening your muscle fibers. To determine your range of motion, first do each exercise with a very light weight, paying careful attention to the movement pattern.

■ Don't rush from one exercise to the next—you'll have better form if you rest slightly between sets.

■ Always allow at least 48 hours for recovery time (one full rest day) between strength workouts. This is how long it takes for your muscles to resynthesize and rebuild.

■ Once 12 repetitions of a strength exercise start to feel easy, increase the weight of each dumbbell by five pounds.

THE ZEN OF STRENGTH TRAINING

Here is what Wayne Westcott has to say about why weight-lifting exercises should always be done slowly and deliberately:

"Fast movements are more dangerous and less effective than slow strength training. Slow movements will produce more tension and force in the muscle, enhancing your strength development.

Exercise 1: Dumbbell Squat (or Leg Extension Machine)

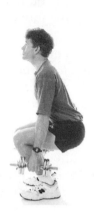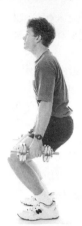

Begin with feet flat on the floor, a shoulder's width apart. Hold the dumbbells at your side, with your arms fully extended. Keeping your head up, your back straight, and your feet flat on the floor, slowly lower your hips until your thighs are parallel to the floor.

Maintaining this "head up, back straight" posture, return to your starting position. Repeat 8 to 12 times.

Exercise 2: Dumbbell Lunge (or Leg Curl Machine)

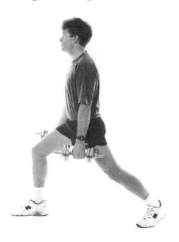

Stand holding both dumbbells, with your arms hanging naturally at your sides and your feet slightly less than a shoulder's width apart. Looking straight ahead, step forward with one leg, keeping your rear leg straight. Your forward leg should be bent, with your knee directly over your ankle. Keeping your weight evenly distributed on both feet, bend your back leg until the knee almost touches the floor. Push off with your front foot, and return to starting position. Do this 8 to 12 times, then switch legs and repeat.

Exercise 3: Dumbbell Bench Press (or Chest Press Machine)

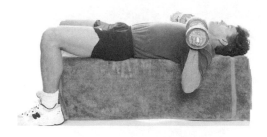

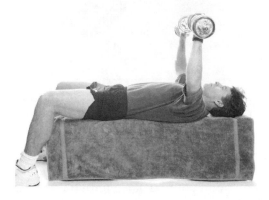

Lie face up on a smooth bench, with your feet flat on the floor. Hold both dumbbells above your chest, with your arms fully extended. Slowly lower the dumbbells to your chest, allowing your elbows to point out to either side. Then slowly press the dumbbells up to starting position, counting "one one thousand, two one thousand," and so on. Repeat 8 to 12 times.

Exercise 4: Bent-over Dumbbell Row (or Lat Pull-down Machine)

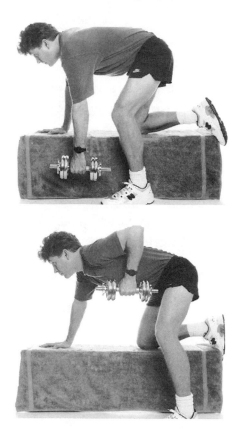

Holding a dumbbell in one hand, place your other, free hand on a bench or chair, so that your back is supported in a horizontal position. Hold the dumbbell so that your arm is fully extended, and slowly pull the dumbbell to your chest, to a count of "one one thousand, two one thousand"—keeping your head up and your back straight. Then slowly lower the dumbbell to starting position, maintaining this same "head up, back straight" posture. Do 8 to 12 repetitions, then switch arms and repeat.

WEEK FOUR

(DAYS 22–28)

Total aerobic time: 2:45 (165 minutes)

Total calories burned: 990 calories if you weigh 165 lbs.; 1145 calories, 190 lbs.; 1320 calories, 220 lbs.

WEEKLY CHECKLIST

☐ Did I do at least 25 minutes of aerobic activity five times this week?

☐ Did I do one long aerobic workout?

☐ Did I make healthy choices in what I did and ate?

DAY	22	23	23
WORKOUT:			
COMMENTS:			
RESTING HR:			

Week Four

GOAL: To complete your initial adjustment to daily aerobic exercise, with a week that includes almost three hours of aerobic training time, including a long workout of 45 minutes.

WEEKLY REPORT: These are the last seven days of the hardest part of your new exercise program, so be sure to get plenty of sleep and nourishment this week. Stick to a moderate pace throughout your workouts, and put in a good effort on your long, three-quarters of an hour session. Congratulate yourself when you hit day 28—you've got your first month under your belt. From here on, your aerobic fitness will rise steadily, and workouts will get easier.

Since this week's Workout Adviser features nutrition, this might be a good time to check out the eating habits of John Jones. John is a creature of habit and tends to eat the same thing for breakfast every weekday morning: two doughnuts, an apple, and a cup of coffee with half-and-half. (On weekends, he'll add scrambled eggs and English muffins.) For lunch during the week, he either goes out to a restaurant with a business associate, or gets a sandwich and a salad at a nearby deli. At home, his wife has been nutrition-

24	25	26	27

conscious for years, cooking with low-fat oil and serving red meat sparingly. John does tend to splurge on ice cream and/or cake for dessert at night, but who can blame him? Outside of that, his diet looks pretty harmless.

But then why were his cholesterol levels so high? A month after his checkup, at his doctor's recommendation, John met with a nutritionist. He was shocked to hear how much saturated fat was in the luncheon meat and salad dressing he ate each day for lunch, and in the ice cream he loved so much after dinner, and in the half-and-half he drank each morning. But he was even more astonished when the nutritionist explained that most of the doughnuts, pies, and cakes he ate were loaded with another, equally dangerous fat: hydrogenated vegetable oil, which has been chemically treated and has been shown to increase dangerous cholesterol levels *and* decrease HDL cholesterol at the same time. These same hydrogenated fats, said the nutrionist, are used to cook food in most fast-food chains—and the fat content of food at many more expensive restaurants isn't any better.

What's a guy to do? In John's case, not all that much. At the advice of the nutritionist, he now adds skim milk to his coffee and carefully buys low-fat doughnuts at a local gourmet food shop before getting on the train each morning. For lunch he now shuns pastrami, ham, and roast beef in favor of chicken, turkey, or tuna salad sandwiches (made with low-fat mayonnaise—he asks to be sure) and salad with low-fat vinaigrette dressing. If he goes out to a restaurant, he'll usually order a poultry or pasta dish with vegetables (no fried potatoes or onions, though), and he checks to be sure the dish is cooked in a low-fat method.

On the weekends, John now eats eggs only one day, and instead of butter he spreads his English muffins with a mixture of half butter half olive oil, which is actually quite delicious. The nighttime ice cream has gone by the wayside, but frozen yogurt and home-made, low-fat cakes and cookies are still on the menu.

With these measures, John has cut his daily fat intake in half. And with a low-fat apple pie cooling on top of the oven, he doesn't really feel he's missing a thing.

Workout Adviser: Fueling the Engine

Contrary to popular belief, there are no special "athletic" nutritional diets. A balanced diet is a balanced diet, whether you're exercising regularly or not. The main difference between the needs of fit and unfit people is that fit people tend to eat more of each nutrient— yet paradoxically, they gain less weight.

That's because exercise helps to fine-tune your appetite mechanism, which tends to switch off when you don't get any exercise. This, together with your higher daily calorie output and increased muscle mass from exercise, makes it much easier to unconsciously eat exactly the right amount of daily calories and avoid the "creeping obesity" that comes from years of eating a few extra calories each day.

One thing recreational athletes *don't* need more of, though, is protein. For optimum muscle growth, the average man needs to eat about four-tenths of a gram of protein per day for every pound he weighs. For a 170-pound man, this comes out to 2 ounces of protein a day—a requirement that goes up only when you do very strenuous exercise. But the average American takes in over 10 ounces of protein a day, mostly from meat and milk—much more protein than you'll ever need, athlete or not.

Another thing that Americans definitely don't need more of is dietary fat. The average U.S. citizen gets over 40 percent of his daily calories from fat—compared to about 10 percent in many Asian countries. Doctors now recommend cutting that figure to between 20 and 30 percent. (For a more detailed discussion of how fats affect your health, see the following section.)

What this leaves, of course, is the athlete's best friend: carbohydrates, especially complex carbohydrates like those found in cereal, fruit, vegetables, pasta, rice, bread, and other grains. Taking in enough carbohydrates is essential when you're exercising, in order to keep your muscles' glycogen stores fully stocked. Moderate exercisers need a diet that's between 50 and 60 percent carbohydrates, to give them about 400 to 500 grams of carbos a day—which is what the typical American already eats.

This prescription changes, though, if you decide to start a heavy aerobic training program, like preparing to run a marathon. In that case, you'll need to eat proportionally more carbohydrates, to make sure you don't deplete your muscles—up to 70 percent of your diet.

For those of us who aren't planning to do the Ironman triathlon, and are already eating more than enough of everything, the best advice is to try to cut back on the fat and boost the complex carbohydrates.

WHY THE PRE-WORKOUT CANDY BAR IS A BIG MISTAKE

Another old exercise myth is the idea that eating something sweet or drinking a sugared sports drink before a workout will give you a boost in energy. But scientific studies have found that athletes who are fed glucose (sugar) before an exercise session actually have *reduced* endurance! This is because the sugar triggers a swift rush of insulin in your body, which causes a *drop* in blood sugar (after a brief rise) and also temporarily blocks your body's ability to burn fats—which are half of your energy supply when you're exercising.

If you do eat something sweet, do it at least three hours before exercising. (This is also the minimum time you should allow for digesting a pre-workout meal.)

The sugar story is different once you're into your workout, however. Studies have shown that drinking a sugary liquid *during* exercise can actually improve your performance, especially during long, intense workouts. The reason for this difference is probably that the hormones released during exercise override your body's insulin response.

Body Maintenance Manual: Eating for a Healthy Body

Sexism can cut both ways. Take the "dumb husband" stereotype when it comes to nutrition. This poor sap was the off-screen star of a recent ad for a line of low-fat cuisine, now being marketed by a well-known weight-loss company. The product is terrific, but the message was rotten: In the commercial, a "nutrition savvy" woman was shown gloating over the fact that her dunce of a husband "still hasn't figured out" that she's switched to a low-fat menu!

Men, it's time to take the nutritional intiative! Learning which foods are bad for you or should be limited—particularly fats—takes only a few minutes. The same goes for understanding about antioxidants—the vitamins in certain vegetables that help fight off disease. It's your body and your health, so why not understand what you're eating and how it affects you?

Cut the Fat, Protect Your Heart

Before you shrug and order a hot dog the next time you're at a baseball game, remember this fact: One million Americans die of heart attacks each year, most of them men, and the biggest single reason for this is that they *ate too much fat.*

Not only that, but a high-fat diet is also directly related to the fat on your abdomen. For one thing, a gram of fat has over twice the calories of a gram of carbohydrates or protein (9 calories per gram, versus 4). And your body is also 10 times more efficient at converting dietary fat into stored body fat than it is at converting carbohydrates, meaning you'll build up fat stores much more readily on a high-fat diet. Finally (strike three!) a high-fat meal eaten within hours after working out appears to blunt your natural metabolic response following exercise, negating the calorie-burning aftereffects of your aerobic training.

These are all great reasons to cut down on fat intake. Yet the average American still gets about 40 percent of his calories from fat!

Part of the problem is that we're naturally geared to crave fat.

MAIN SOURCES OF FAT IN THE AMERICAN DIET

Cooking fats and oils (used in fried and sautéed foods, and baked goods)	36 percent
Meat, poultry, and fish	35 percent
Milk, cheese, and cream	14 percent
Butter	5 percent
Eggs	4 percent

In times of famine, our super-efficiency at storing fat calories is a vital survival tool. Even in the modern world, you need *some* fat in your diet—just less than you're probably getting now.

The U.S. Department of Agriculture is now advising people to cut their fat intake to less than 30 percent of their total daily calories. Some doctors are urging that an even lower standard be set—around 20 percent of total calories (about 55 grams of fat per day, for the average man).

But just as important, scientists are getting better at distinguishing which types of fat are most dangerous for your heart and arteries and which fats can be eaten without worrying.

Here's a rundown on who the bad guys and the good guys are:

The Bad Guys

Saturated Fats

They're called saturated because these fat molecules are as chockful of bonded hydrogen atoms as they possibly could be. All these chemical bonds mean that saturated fats are greasy to the touch and are usually solid at room temperature. Butter, lard, and coconut oil are examples of almost pure saturated fats. Meat—especially processed meat, like baloney or hot dogs—is also high in saturated fat, and so is whole milk, cream, and cheese.

THEIR CRIME: Saturated fats significantly raise the level of low-density lipoprotein (LDL) cholesterol in the bloodstream. LDL cholesterol is the molecule that deposits fat on your coronary artery walls, leading eventually to a narrowing of these arteries—a recipe for a heart attack. Besides aiding and abetting these villains, saturated fats also cause your blood to clot more easily—increasing the chances of a clot in your heart, which could cause a heart attack, or in your brain, where a clot could trigger a stroke.

Diets high in these nutritional undesirables have also been associated with increased rates of breast cancer and colon cancer—although the evidence here is less than airtight. An abundance of saturated fats in your gut and your bloodstream also encourages the bad behavior of our second-most-wanted criminal: hydrogenated fats.

Hydrogenated Fats

These are fats that start out as mainly unsaturated fats, which are more or less neutral, as far as your heart is concerned. But they've been treated chemically to allow more hydrogen atoms to bond to each molecule—effectively turning them into saturated fats. As you might guess, that process turns liquid vegetable fat into slippery, semisolid vegetable shortening, to be used in frying fast food, baked into commercial pies, breads, cookies, and cakes, and served up as margarine.

Mass manufacturers like to use hydrogenated fats because they're convenient, easy to use and ship, and last longer than vegetable oils. A number of years ago, there was also a belief that hydrogenated fats were better for your heart than traditional saturated fats. That's why margarine was touted as a healthy substitute for butter. Today, we know that these safety claims simply aren't true.

THEIR CRIME: Hydrogenated vegetable oils have been shown to raise LDL cholesterol in your bloodstream, *and* lower the levels of HDL cholesterol—the "good" cholesterol that works to remove LDL from your arteries. Since the ratio of HDL to total cholesterol is the most accurate predictor of heart disease, these fats affect your cholesterol levels in the worst possible way.

Gram for gram, hydrogenated fats are now considered just as dangerous as saturated fats, if eaten in excess. And because they're so prevalent in fast-food and commercial baked goods (just check any package in the supermarket), these fats are often "hidden" in your daily diet and less easy to spot and avoid than true saturated fats are.

Cholesterol

This molecule is not technically a fat, but it acts like one. It's primarily found in egg yolks, shellfish, red meat, and dairy products.

THE CRIME: Like saturated fats, dietary cholesterol tends to raise LDL cholesterol levels in the bloodstream—about 6 percent, on average, if you eat two eggs a day. This effect varies widely from person to person, however.

ON THE FENCE

Polyunsaturated Fats

These are fats with two or more double hydrogen bonds, which means they aren't saturated with hydrogen. This makes them liquid at room temperature. Safflower oil, corn oil, soybean oil, and sunflower oil all contain mostly polyunsaturated fat.

SUSPICIOUS ACTIVITIES: These polyunsaturated vegetable oils appear to lower dangerous LDL cholesterol in the bloodstream a bit—which is good—but they *also* lower protective HDL cholesterol levels—which is bad. Current thinking is that these fats are okay in small quantities—7 percent or less of your total calories.

THE GOOD GUYS

Monounsaturated Fats

These health-abiding characters have one double bond of hydrogen, which is what gives them their name. Like the polyunsaturates, these fats are liquid at room temperature. Olive oil, canola oil, and peanut oil all contain mostly monounsaturated fats.

HONORS AWARDED: Basically these are the safest fats to eat, since they don't affect blood cholesterol or clotting in any significant way. These fats, particularly olive oil and canola oil, are by far the healthiest cooking oils to use for frying or baking.

Omega 3 Oils

These fatty oils are polyunsaturated fats, but they're found not in vegetables, but in cold-water fish—particularly tuna, sardines, mackerel, and herring.

HONORS AWARDED: Regular intake of omega 3 oils appears to improve the blood's cholesterol profile and lower heart attack risk. Scientists speculate this may be due to some anticlotting effect.

ANTIOXIDANTS: THE FOUNTAIN OF YOUTH

Eat your vegetables!

Of all the advice your mother ever gave you, this might have been the most farsighted of all. Scientists are just now unravelling the reason vitamin-rich fruits and vegetables are so health promoting. The answer is: antioxidants.

To put it simply, the cells in your body tend to "rust," or oxidize, the same way metal rusts, fruit turns brown, and oil becomes rancid. This rusting is caused by particles called free radicals. To keep the process from getting out of control, your body employs a variety of scavenger enzymes called antioxidants, which patrol your body's cells, neutralizing any free radicals they happen to bump into.

Some scientists believe that slowing down this cellular oxidation may be the key to stopping the aging process—and that keeping your body supplied with plenty of antioxidants could be one step in that direction.

That's all just speculation at this point, but high levels of certain antioxidants *have* been shown to protect people from getting illnesses like cancer, coronary artery disease, cataracts, and Parkinson's disease. The exact mechanism of these enzymes isn't yet known: For one thing, antioxidants seem to reinforce each other, which means that even the hundreds of very rare antioxidants may have important roles.

Antioxidants fall into several categories, including some enzymes that are manufactured naturally by our bodies, and some that we get from our diet—either from vegetables or in vitamin supplements.

Here are the major dietary antioxidants and the diseases they protect against:

Vitamin E

Vitamin E has been shown to protect against heart disease (by preventing plaque buildup in the arteries), and also inhibits blood clotting (giving protection against a heart attack). It's also been linked to lower levels of lung cancer and breast cancer and may help delay the progress of degenerative nerve diseases like Parkinson's and Alzheimer's.

In addition, there's evidence that high levels of Vitamin E in your body can help prevent exercise-related muscle soreness and damage and can help older people adapt more quickly to the stress of exercise. Vitamin E is fat-soluble, meaning it goes into many body tissues and isn't easily excreted. For this reason, large doses of Vitamin E may be toxic.

SOURCES: Vegetable oils, eggs, fish, green leafy vegetables, whole grains, dried beans.

Vitamin C

Vitamin C appears to enhance the immune system and has been linked to reduced risk of stomach and colon cancer. It also appears to inhibit blood clotting (giving protection against a heart attack). In addition, Vitamin C enhances the action of Vitamin E by recycling spent Vitamin E molecules.

SOURCES: Citrus fruits, tomatoes, broccoli, cabbage, cauliflower, green peppers, strawberries, potatoes.

Beta-carotene

This antioxidant protects against lung cancer, improves immune response, and stimulates Vitamin A activity. Beta-carotene has also slowed the growth of cancer cells in animals. Very high levels of beta-carotene (like those produced by some supplements) may actually be harmful, however, by interfering with the digestion of other nutrients.

SOURCES: Broccoli, cantaloupe, carrots.

Lycopene

Technically a phytochemical (which is similar to an antioxidant), lycopene protects against colon and bladder cancer and has recently been shown to be potent in protecting against cardiovascular disease. Lycopene has also slowed the growth of cancer cells in animals.

SOURCES: Tomatoes and tomato products.

Lutein

This protects against lung cancer and also appears to protect against macular degeneration—a leading cause of blindness in older adults.

SOURCES: Broccoli, spinach, collard greens.

Alpha-carotene

Alpha-carotene increases Vitamin A activity, protects against lung cancer, and improves the immune response. It has also been shown to slow the growth of cancer cells in animals.

SOURCE: Carrots.

Should You Take Supplements?

The standard advice of nutritionists and doctors has always been that the average U.S. diet is so rich in vitamins, Americans don't really need vitamin and mineral supplements except in cases where a specific deficiency is diagnosed.

Now with new evidence that high levels of antioxidants can protect against cancer and heart disease, there's been a surge of interest in supplements, especially of Vitamins E, C, and beta-carotene. Several B vitamins have also been shown to be important in protecting against heart disease:

Folic acid (found in leafy green vegetables, organ meats, non-leafy vegetables, apples, bread, nuts, and beans)

Vitamin B_6 (found in meat, poultry, and fish, whole grains, eggs and dairy products, and most fruits and vegetables)

Vitamin B_{12} (found in beef, pork, lamb, poultry, fish, eggs, milk, and milk products)

The mainstream thinking now seems to be that supplements are okay, as long as they're in the range of the standard minimum daily requirements. Megadoses of vitamins can be worse than nothing at all: Vitamin E can be toxic in high levels, and large doses of beta-carotene actually *increased* the risk of lung cancer in one study of male smokers!

Scientists speculate that high doses of a single antioxidant may "push out" other key nutrients. There are literally thousands of trace antioxidants and related phytochemicals in vegetables, which work together in ways that aren't yet understood. This is an excellent reason to get your main supply of antioxidants from food instead of from a vitamin capsule: It'll be decades before any supplements can match the complex mix of enzymes found in one piece of broccoli!

"Until we identify the protective entities in fruits and vegetables, we can't encapsulate them in a pill," says Dr. Regina Ziegler, a scientist at the National Cancer Institute in Maryland. "At this point, the best advice to the public is to increase their intake of fruits and vegetables."

TEN TIPS FOR A LOW-FAT DIET

1. Avoid all processed meats: baloney, salami, pepperoni, hot dogs, and pâté.

2. Try to keep the red meat you eat to a minimum, and choose lean cuts. For protein, substitute poultry or fish for red meat whenever possible, or go vegetarian with a combination of a grain and a legume (dried or canned beans)—for example a rice and bean casserole. A bit of cheese or other dairy product will enhance this protein package even more.

3. Avoid whole milk, whole cheese, and ice cream. Substitute low-fat milk (1 percent or skim), low-fat cheese, and frozen yogurt.

4. Do all home cooking with olive oil, canola oil, sesame seed oil, or some other monounsaturated fat.

5. Limit yourself to four or less whole eggs a week. After that, use just the egg whites (separating out the yolk).

6. Instead of butter (which is mostly saturated fat) or margarine (which is hydrogenated fat), try using a mixture of half butter and half olive oil. Stir together until they become semiliquid, then put into the refrigerator to harden.

7. Check any baked goods you buy for hydrogenated fat content. Try to select non-fat or low-fat bread, doughnuts, cakes, etc.

8. Avoid eating all fast food (i.e., burgers, french fries, fried chicken, burritos) unless the restaurant offers a specific low-fat menu. Most fast-food chains cook these foods in hydrogenated fats, which lower your good (HDL) cholesterol and raise levels of dangerous (LDL) cholesterol.

9. Avoid eating sugar-rich foods. Sugar is a "simple" carbohydrate, easily digested, and it will send your insulin levels soaring—which prevents your muscles from burning fat as fuel. Stick to "complex" carbohydrates like pasta, vegetables, fruit, and whole grains like rice, wheat, or corn.

10. Keep a weather eye out for fat in all snack foods, especially potato chips and other greasy foods (remember, a greasy texture is the hallmark of saturated fat). Become a label-reader. There's usually a low-fat alternative for any favorite food. Even Hollywood's getting the word: Many movie theaters now sell popcorn with canola oil—a much healthier (monounsaturated) alternative to the butter (saturated fat) we're used to dosing ourselves with.

WEEK FIVE

(DAYS 29–35)

Two 30-minute workouts
Three 45-minute workouts
(two strength workouts)

Total aerobic time: 3:15 (195 minutes)

Total calories burned: 1170 calories if you weigh 165 lbs.; 1365 calories, 190 lbs.; 1560 calories, 220 lbs.

WEEKLY CHECKLIST

☐ Did I do at least 30 minutes of aerobic activity five times this week?

☐ Did I do one long aerobic workout?

☐ Did I make healthy choices in what I did and ate?

DAY	29	30	31
WORKOUT:			
COMMENTS:			
RESTING HR:			

WEEK FIVE

GOAL: To begin a month of steady fitness building, while maintaining a workload of three-plus hours of aerobic training per week.

WEEKLY REPORT: This is the time to keep the faith: The most stressful part of getting in shape is now behind you. You can expect to feel stronger and fitter in each week of this next phase. Maintain an easy-to-moderate pace in workouts this week, as your weekly training load creeps up by another half hour, to 195 minutes. Concentrate on making a reasonable schedule, then sticking to it. There's no long workout planned for this week.

By now you've been doing workouts of 30 minutes or more for several weeks, and you should be starting to feel your own natural rhythm in these workouts: beginning slowly, then picking up the pace according to your own internal clock, until you hit a smooth plateau of steady walking, cycling, or swimming that takes you enjoyably through the half-hour mark and beyond. Although some guys like to finish strong, with a burst of effort toward the end

32	33	34	35

of the workout, it's not really necessary—the benefits come throughout your workout, just by holding that steady, relaxed pace.

The first month of regular exercise is a time of physical adjustment, but it's also a shakedown cruise—an opportunity to sort out how your exercise plan fits into your daily life. John Jones has come to a few realizations. One thing he's found is that getting two workouts in every weekend was essential for him, because of time demands during the work week. Another discovery he's made is that he likes cycling better than walking. He's now settled on cycling Saturdays and Sundays, racketball on Wednesdays, and walking twice a week, usually Tuesday and Friday mornings, when he puts in 30 minutes before going to the office. If he's pressed for time, he divides these walking workouts in half—15 minutes in the morning, and 15 minutes walking home from the train in the evening. On these days, he wears a pair of walking shoes to work (a popular brand designed to look like dress shoes—John doesn't like to stand out in the crowd) and then changes into an extra pair of wingtips he keeps at the office.

This plan seems to fit John's life-style perfectly, and he's already feeling stronger and trimmer, even if there's no real evidence on the bathroom scale yet (he's actually lost about two pounds—representing a small but very real reduction in body fat).

Workout Adviser: Logistical Planning

To make your exercise plan effective, you've got to be like a general, marshalling your time and energy to maximum advantage. The most important factor is a regular exercise location. It may be your neighborhood, a local park or schoolyard, a health club, a high school pool, or a walking track at a gym. If you're cycling for fitness, this means establishing a regular route or a short loop that you can repeat several times.

This locale should be a place you feel secure, and it should be a route that has little or no traffic. It should also be a location you have easy access to. If you live in a neighborhood with sidewalks, you've got yourself an ideal walking area.

A regular workout place takes the guesswork out of scheduling. You can always add new locales as you go along.

As for when to work out, the answer is, whenever you can. Early morning is a favorite time for many people, especially cyclists, who can steal a march on the day's auto traffic. Just give yourself an extra few minutes of puttering around before you start off, to give your body a chance to shake off the effects of sleep. For commuters, walking or cycling to their train or bus stop is a perfect aerobic opportunity. If you live close to your workplace, cycle all the way and get a bonus workout coming home. (Millions of Chinese commuters do it every day.)

A lunch break can work, too, if you have enough time and access to a shower. For walkers who don't sweat too heavily, lunchtime is ideal. (Lunchtimers should consider buying an athletic bag to carry their exercise shoes in.) But after-work aerobics seems to be the favorite time slot for most Americans: It's a good time to blow off some steam, there's less time pressure, and the mid-to-late afternoon is also when your physical biorhythms are peaking.

Structuring Your Workouts

The Fit Again program recommends using a wristwatch to gauge your aerobic workouts by time, rather than trying to measure the distance you're covering. Most people settle quickly into a steady walking pace somewhere between three and four miles in an hour of steady walking—a mile every 15 to 20 minutes. By this estimate, a half-hour of walking is about two miles, 45 minutes is about three miles, and so on.

How do you know how long you've been working out? If you're on a treadmill in a club or swimming in a pool, there's probably a clock on the wall; otherwise your best bet is to purchase an inexpensive sports watch. When you're walking or cycling in unfamiliar surroundings, simply head back toward your starting point when you hit the halfway time point in your workout. If you have a regular walking or biking route, you'll soon get a sense of how long it takes to cover the distance, and you won't need to rely on your watch as much.

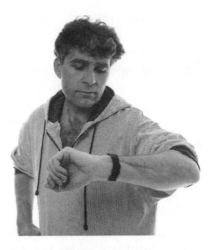

The Fit Again program recommends measuring your workouts by elapsed time. You can buy a sports watch for under $20.

As you get more accustomed to planning exercise slots in your week, you should also be experimenting with different workout formulas that help make exercise "do-able." If you can't get a full workout in, don't panic: Aerobic training is cumulative, which lets you add up the minutes of exercise you get throughout the day. Here are some variations on the basic workout theme:

- You can slice a day's workout in half, putting in part of a workout in the morning, the other part in the evening.
- You can stop in the middle of a workout for a stretching or strength training session, before continuing.
- If you only have small openings in your schedule and find longer workouts impossible, go to a fall-back plan of 30 aerobic minutes per day, and try to get in six or seven days of exercise a week.
- You can mix and match various aerobic activities in 10- or 15-minute segments: for example, 15 minutes on a stationary bike,

15 minutes on a stair-climbing machine, and 15 minutes of walking.

■ You can also vary your workouts from day to day and from week to week. One good idea is to alternate days of hard effort and days of easier effort. Many athletes also try to alternate "hard" weeks and "easier" weeks.

As you get more experienced and fit, you'll find that shaping a workout is really an art form. The key is to keep coming up with variations that will keep your body challenged and your mind sharp and refreshed.

Body Maintenance Manual: Six Anti-aging Stretches

Stretching is a personal matter—some guys get a lot out of it, others don't. When you're involved in an aerobic/strength program, stretching isn't a top priority, since you'll tend to use only a limited range of motion in your aerobic exercise. Increasing your flexibility is much more important when you're preparing for sports like golf, softball, tennis, or touch football, where you'll be using a much larger range of motion, and stressing your joints and muscles more.

On the other hand, time and gravity naturally cause tightness in some areas, if they're not stretched from time to time. This is especially true with your hamstrings, your lower back, and your hips. Repetitive exercise like walking, cycling, or running can contribute to this problem. The repeated motion of aerobic exercise is great for your metabolism and your heart, but it won't change the way your muscles relate to each other. Muscles that are weak and tight at age 25 tend to be weak and tight at age 45, if you don't do specific exercises for them.

In fact, most muscle imbalances tend to get *worse* over time, affecting your posture and your biomechanical efficiency. Muscles always work in paired groupings—one muscle group relaxes and stretches while the opposing group contracts. When you crouch down, for instance, your hamstrings contract, while the muscles in the front of your thigh relax and lengthen. When you stand up, the reverse happens.

But if a muscle is tight, it prevents its opposing number from contracting as efficiently as it could. (For example, tight hamstrings will rob your legs of power when you walk.) Tight muscles also tend to be chronically weak, forcing nearby muscles to take up the strain when work is required.

This syndrome is especially common in people who have recurring back pain. Their hamstrings and lower backs tend to be weak and tight, causing the pelvis to tilt forward. This transfers weight to inappropriate back muscles, which eventually tire out and go into spasm, causing a back ache.

If you should have the misfortune to suffer any kind of chronic pain, such as a sore back, then stretching turns into a necessity. Overuse injuries are usually a sign of tight or weak muscles, and a stretching program is an important part of the rehabilitation process. (The hamstring stretch and hip flexor stretch, both shown below, are especially effective for keeping your back healthy and pain-free.)

The following stretches work specifically on the areas that tend to get tighter as you get older: your calf muscles, your hamstrings, your hip flexors (which move your upper thigh forward at the hip), your lower back, your chest muscles, and finally your neck.

You'll certainly find them relaxing. You might also find that they help your posture and walking stride—especially the calf, hamstring, and lower-back stretches. Many exercisers have discovered that stretching every day after working out adds an extra ease and fluidity to their aerobic activities and helps keep soreness away.

Note: When you do a stretching exercise, you're not really stretching your muscles themselves—you're actually tugging and lengthening the microscopic elastic wrappings *around* your muscle fibers. These wrappings are at their most stretchable when your muscles are *fully warmed up,* in the middle or end of an aerobic workout. That's when any serious stretching should take place. Any stretching you do *before* your workout should be light and brief, just enough to limber up a little. The real warm-up for your muscles is the workout itself.

The Rules of Stretching

- All stretching movements should be smooth and gradual. Never bounce or force a stretch—you can injure a muscle or tendon that way.
- Stretch within five to ten minutes after finishing your workout, while your muscles are still warm (or take a midway break in your workout for a stretching session).
- Relax and hold each stretch for at least 15 seconds, at a point where you feel a pleasant tension in the muscle groups being stretched. Concentrate on this pleasant sensation and feel your muscles gradually lengthen.
- Don't hold your breath as you feel the stretch in your muscles; instead, breathe easily in and out through your nostrils, keep your neck and shoulder relaxed, and round, don't arch, your back.
- *Never* do any stretching movement that causes pain or discomfort.

Six Anti-aging Stretches

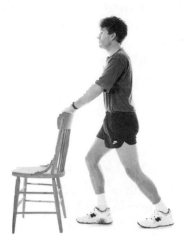

1. CALF-ACHILLES STRETCH.   This stretch can be done with your hands on hips, or pushing against a wall for support.

Stand comfortably with your feet a few inches apart. Step with your right foot, so that your toes are slightly behind your left heel. Bend both knees slightly, keeping your feet flat on the floor and your weight over your right foot. Go down slowly, until you feel a stretch in your right Achilles tendon (running down the back of your calf and heel). Hold for 15 to 30 seconds. Repeat with legs reversed.

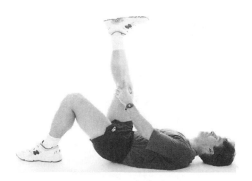

2. HAMSTRING STRETCH.   Lie on your back and bend your left leg, keeping your left foot flat on the floor. Keeping your right leg straight (but not locking your knee), lift it from the hip until you feel a gentle stretch in your right hamstring (running down the back of your thigh). If you want, you can clasp your hands behind your right knee to assist in the stretch. Hold for 15 to 30 seconds, then repeat with legs reversed.

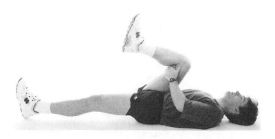

3. LOWER BACK STRETCH.   Lie on your back with your legs extended. Bend your right leg, and clasp your hands behind your right knee. Then pull your right knee toward your chest, keeping your left leg very straight, and hold it for 15 to 30 seconds. Repeat with your left leg, then with both legs together.

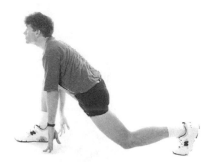

4. HIP FLEXOR STRETCH.   Kneeling with your left knee resting on the floor, move your right leg forward so your right foot is flat on the ground and your right knee is directly over your right ankle. Holding that position, gently lower your left hip toward the ground. A slight downward movement should produce a stretching sensation in the front of your left hip. Hold for 15 to 30 seconds, then repeat with legs reversed.

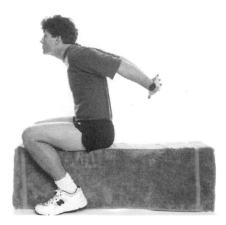

5. CHEST STRETCH.   This stretch can be done while you're standing or sitting. Lace your fingers behind your back, so your palms are facing in toward your spine. Raise your hands up toward the ceiling until you feel a stretching sensation in the front of your chest. Don't arch your back, and be sure to keep your neck in a relaxed, neutral position. Hold for 15 to 30 seconds.

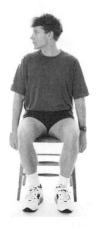

6. NECK STRETCH.   Sit comfortably in a chair. Shrug your shoulders and then relax them slowly. Do this several times. Next, inhale deeply and drop your chin towards your chest. Exhale and return to starting position. Do this several times. Finally, sit with your chin tucked in slightly and inhale deeply, turning your head to the left as far as it will comfortably go. Exhale and return to your starting position, then repeat the stretch to the right side, using the same breathing pattern. Do this several times.

WEEK SIX

(DAYS 36–42)

Two 30-minute workouts
Two 45-minute workouts
One 60-minute workout
(two strength workouts)

Total aerobic time: 3:30 (210 minutes)

Total calories burned: 1260 calories if you weigh 165 lbs.; 1470 calories, 190 lbs.; 1680 calories, 220 lbs.

WEEKLY CHECKLIST

☐ Did I do at least 30 minutes of aerobic activity five times this week?

☐ Did I get in one long aerobic workout?

☐ Did I make healthy choices in what I did and ate?

DAY	36	37	38
WORKOUT: **COMMENTS:**			
RESTING HR:			

Week Six

GOAL: To achieve your full workload goal of three-and-a-half hours' aerobic training, with one long workout of 60 minutes.

STATUS REPORT: Pace should be moderate this week. Your short workouts should start feeling much easier at this point. Concentrate on pacing yourself carefully in your 60-minute session.

The big news this week, if you're following this program to the letter, is a full one hour of aerobic activity. The jump from a 45-minute walk to a 60-minute walk looks small on paper, but in reality you're making significantly more demands on your muscles when you keep moving for an entire hour. For one thing, you'll dip slightly into your muscles' stores of sugar (technically known as glycogen), which exist for just these kinds of adventures. As a result, you might feel a little more fatigued the next day, and you'll almost certainly crave more carbohydrates (grains, fruits, and vegetables) to replenish your glycogen supplies.

The second month of your program is also a time when some physical changes should be visible—while you may not have lost

39	40	41	42

many pounds on the scale, you may find yourself tightening your belt an extra notch, a sign that you've been trading fat in for muscle. John Jones has actually been getting comments from people, like "Have you lost weight?" to which he answers, "Not really," and "Are you working out?" to which he answers, "Yeah, when I can find the time."

In fact, he has been very conscientious about making time for his exercise, taking maximum advantage of his weekends and commuting hours. The hardest part for John, as an ex-jock, is accepting the fact that daily aerobic workouts are really exercise—even though there's no huffing, no blood-curdling grunts, and no banging against walls. The thing is, John's already feeling almost as fit as he did in his wall-banging days; and he's starting to believe there might be something to this aerobic stuff after all.

Workout Adviser: Why Exercise Beats Dieting

Here's some news that will come as a shock to anyone who's ever said, "I really shouldn't be eating this." Doctors are now finding evidence that it *really doesn't matter* whether or not you eat that extra dessert—and that overweight people may not be overeating at all, but simply underexercising!

A new study at Rockefeller University in New York City, published early in 1995, showed that when people intentionally ate more food than usual (consuming 5,000 to 6,000 calories a day), they gained weight—up to 10 percent of their original body weight. But the big surprise was that their muscle metabolisms sped up too! As a result, the overeaters burned more calories, both at rest and when they moved about. After the special diet was stopped and they started eating as much as they felt like, these people returned to their starting weights, and their metabolisms returned to normal.

This was true both for people who were overweight and people who weren't. When the subjects went on a very restrictive diet of 800 calories a day and *lost* weight, the reverse happened: Their muscles slowed down, so that the dieters were burning fewer calories, even during exercise. Once the diet period ended and the subjects could eat freely, both groups rebounded to their starting weights—and their muscle metabolisms returned to normal.

What this indicates, says Dr. Jules Hirsch, the senior author of the study, is that being overweight is not an eating disorder, but "an eating order." In other words, your body will automatically work to keep your fat levels right where they are, by revving your muscles when you overeat and slowing them down if you go on a diet. And in fact, long-term studies show that most Americans put on weight very slowly, gaining an average of 10 percent in body weight over 20 years. That works out to only a few excess calories a day.

What pushes people's fat levels slowly upward is the combination of plenty of available food and *a steady decline in muscle mass and muscle activity* over the years. Doctors now believe that encouraging your muscles to burn more calories is the key to lowering your body fat and achieving a new, leaner state of equilibrium.

Regular exercise holds down fat levels in four ways:

1. It burns a few extra hundred calories a day, tipping your daily energy balance slightly in the direction of weight loss.
2. It increases your muscle mass, especially if you do some strength training along with your aerobics. To maintain this new lean tissue, your body will divert calories that would have gone to maintaining your fat stores.
3. Exercise stimulates your muscles to burn a greater proportion of the fat you eat (which is stored as body fat more easily than carbohydrates are).
4. If you're on a diet, regular exercise will help prevent the metabolic slowdown in your muscles that otherwise occurs when you reduce your normal food intake.

With the Fit Again program you can actually turn back the clock, by restoring a foundation of fit muscle tissue that will work as a metabolic anchor, drawing off hundreds of calories a day that would otherwise get stored as fat. This daily "calorie drain" is enough to tip your energy balance, enabling you to start developing a leaner, meaner physique.

It's the little secret that the diet centers don't want you to know: Instead of worrying about how many calories you took in, you're better off counting how many calories you *burned* in physical activity, aiming for a few hundred "aerobic calories" each day.

"The key thing is to use the muscles," said another of the Rockefeller researchers when the landmark study was published. "I'm speaking from personal experience," he added. "I bought a car five years ago, and gained 30 pounds."

The Myth of the "Fat-burning Zone"

You may have heard that exercising at a slower rate will burn fat "better" than exercising at a vigorous pace. Like most popular myths, this one is a half-truth at best. During all but the most intense types of exercise, your body will burn carbohydrates and fats in about a 50–50 ratio. (As you get in better shape, the proportion of fat being burned goes up slightly, thanks to increases in muscle enzymes.)

The idea that there's a special fat-burning "zone" stems from the fact that the proportion of fat burned goes down slightly as your muscles work harder, because they begin to draw on their glucose reserves, which are pure carbohydrate. But this drop is small—and since *total* calories burned goes up when you work harder, you'll burn more total fat in a brisk walk than a slow one if you're covering the same distance.

A better argument for easing up on the pace is to allow your body to exercise for a longer time. When it comes to the length of your workout, there *is* a fat-burning zone. In fact there are two of them. The first is between 45 and 60 minutes—enough time to get your metabolism into full fat-burning mode. That's why the Fit Again program favors three workouts of 45 minutes or longer.

The second, even more effective, fat-burning zone starts once you pass the hour mark in your workout. At this point, your muscle glycogen is somewhat depleted, and the percentage of fat burned starts to rise steadily, for as long as you continue.

This is one reason why the Fit Again program recommends one long workout each week. Another reason is that long workouts are especially good for promoting the growth of new capillaries— the tiny blood vessels that ferry blood to your working muscles. Capillary growth is one of the most durable benefits of exercise. You'll continue to grow new capillaries for as long as you do aerobic exercise, and they'll persist for quite a while even if you stop exercising. (Most of your short-term fitness would vanish in just a few weeks if you returned to "couch potato" status.)

Body Maintenance Manual: Sharpening Your Balance

You probably haven't thought about your balance too much since the last time you walked on an icy sidewalk. But a growing number of sports trainers are now using balance drills as a secret weapon to improve athletic performance. Walking and running really involve balancing on one leg, then the other. The more you can enhance your balance, the more controlled and fluid your movements will be.

Every time you stand upright, it's actually a miracle of coordination: Your postural muscles are working constantly to adjust your body position, using feedback from your vision, the nerves in your feet and joints, and also a special mechanism in your inner ear, which tells your brain how your head is positioned. If your nervous system is out of whack—when you've gotten a bump on the head, for example, or had too much alcohol to drink—your balance will be poor, no matter how strong and fit your legs are.

These cueing systems work in concert; it's hard to notice any single component until it's missing, especially your vision. To prove this to yourself, try balancing on your toes, then close your eyes and continue balancing. You'll find it's not too easy without your eyesight feeding helpful corrective signals to your brain and your postural muscles!

Improving your balance is really like playing a musical instrument. It's a neurological skill that takes time for your body to pick up. Some parts of your nervous system adjust faster than others; you'll feel a rolling motion under your feet if you come back on land after just a few hours on an ocean vessel, for example, but it takes years of such adaptation to truly get your sea legs.

One of the best ways to improve your balance on dry land is simply to move about. Being sedentary for even a few hours is enough to temporarily affect your balance, which is why you may feel slightly unsteady when you first step out of bed.

To sharpen your balance further, you need to challenge your balancing skills by withdrawing some of the cues you're used to using, like your vision (by doing balance drills with your eyes closed), or the helpful "shifting" of your weight from one foot to the other (by standing on one foot).

With several days of practice, these drills will create new neural pathways and additional muscle fibers will be stimulated. You'll quickly find yourself moving with a new sense of ease and coordination.

The following exercises are adapted from the "Spring into Action" program developed by Dr. Miriam Nelson of Tufts University. They are divided into two categories: standing drills and walking drills. Practice these exercise daily, and you can expect some clear improvement in your balance after just two weeks—and significant gains after one month.

Standing Exercises

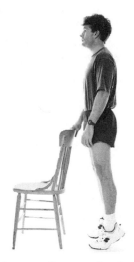

1. TOE STAND.   Stand about a foot and a half from a countertop or wall, with your feet at shoulder width. With one palm flat on the wall for support, raise up as high as you can onto the balls of your feet. Hold for 10 seconds, trying to stand as still as possible. Repeat five times.

Progression: Level one—use one hand to steady yourself. Level two—use no hands unless you lose your balance. Level three—eyes closed, use no hands unless you lose your balance.

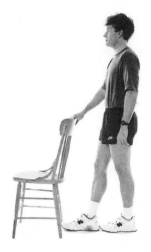

2. TANDEM STAND.   Stand about a foot and a half from a counter-top or wall. With one palm flat on the wall for support, place one foot directly in front of the other, so they're just touching heel-to-toe. Hold for 10 seconds, standing as still as possible and without moving your feet. Repeat five times.

Progression: Level one—use one hand for support. Level two—no hands. Level three—eyes closed, no hands.

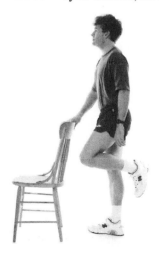

3. ONE-LEGGED STAND.   Stand about a foot and a half away from a countertop or wall. With one palm flat on the wall for support, slowly lift one leg off the floor while balancing on the other leg. Hold for 10 seconds, trying to stand as still as possible and without moving the foot you're standing on. Repeat five times with each leg.

Progression: Level one—use one hand for support. Level two—no hands. Level three—eyes closed, no hands.

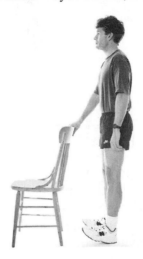

4. HEEL STAND.　　Stand about a foot and a half away from a counter top or wall, with your feet at shoulder width. With one palm flat on the wall for support, raise yourself up as high as you can onto the heels of your feet. Hold this heel stand for 10 seconds, trying to stand as still as possible. Repeat five times.

Progression: Level one—use one hand for support. Level two—no hands. Level three—eyes closed, no hands.

Walking Exercises

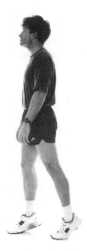

1. TOE WALK. Stand at one end of a 10-foot hallway, an arm's length away from the side wall. Slowly raise up as high as you can onto the balls of your feet. Walk down the hall on your toes, then return to normal standing. Repeat five times.

　　　Progression: Level one—use one hand to touch the wall for balance. Level two—use no hands unless you lose your balance.

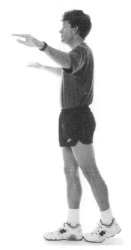

2. TANDEM FORWARD WALK. Stand at one end of a ten-foot hallway, an arm's length away from the side wall. Place one foot in front of the other, so that they just touch heel-to-toe. Walk slowly down the hall, stepping in this same heel-to-toe manner. Repeat five times.

Progression: Level one—use one hand for balance. Level two—no hands.

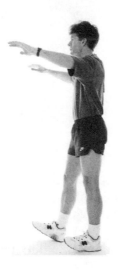

3. HEEL WALK.   Stand at one end of a ten-foot hallway, an arm's length from the side wall. Slowly raise up as high as you can onto your heels, and walk slowly down the hall maintaining this same foot position. Repeat five times.

Progression: Level one—use one hand for balance. Level two—no hands.

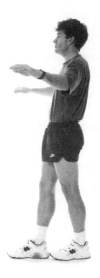

4. TANDEM BACKWARD WALK. Stand at one end of a 10-foot hall-way, an arm's length from the side wall. Turn around, so your back points down the empty hall, and place one foot in back of the other, heel-to-toe. Slowly walk backwards down the hall, stepping in this same heel-to-toe manner. Repeat five times.

Progression: Level one—use one hand for balance. Level two—no hands.

WEEK SEVEN

(DAYS 43–49)

TWO 30-MINUTE WORKOUTS
TWO 45-MINUTE WORKOUTS
ONE 60-MINUTE WORKOUT
(TWO STRENGTH WORKOUTS)

Total aerobic time: 3:30 (210 minutes)

Total calories burned: 1260 calories if you weigh 165 lbs.; 1470 calories, 190 lbs.; 1680 calories, 220 lbs.

WEEKLY CHECKLIST

☐ Did I do at least 30 minutes of aerobic activity five times this week?

☐ Did I do one long aerobic workout?

☐ Did I make healthy choices in what I did and ate?

DAY	43	44	45
WORKOUT: COMMENTS:			
RESTING HR:			

WEEK SEVEN

GOAL: To complete a second week at your full aerobic training load of three-and-a-half hours.

WEEKLY REPORT: Improvements in your muscles' aerobic capacity are now happening at top speed. Muscle enzyme levels will continue to climb steadily at this point, and the size of your slow-twitch (aerobic) muscle fibers will continue to grow slightly over the next few weeks, before levelling off. (If you're also following the weight-lifting program, your fast-twitch, or nonaerobic, fibers will continue to enlarge over the months ahead.)

With your VO_2 max also climbing during this month, you should expect each week to feel easier than the one before. You should also begin to see a steady, gradual decline in your resting heart rate.

The Workout Adviser topic this week is about finding other people to exercise with. John Jones is lucky to have some built-in exercise partners: his mid-week racketball buddies, and his cycling

46	47	48	49

spouse, who has helped him stick to his schedule on the weekends. John and his wife have also discovered an informal local cycling club that has group rides every Saturday morning—8 A.M. for the competitive riders in the group, and a more casual 9 A.M. workout for cyclists like the Joneses, who don't want to go too fast or long. This week was the first time John and his wife rode with the pack. They both found they liked the social atmosphere and also enjoyed the physical feeling of being swept along by the group's enthusiasm.

For his morning walks, John has found he likes to go it alone. He enjoys the chance to think and to watch the city wake up around him. This week, he ran into a woman from his office, who was breathless after rushing from a workout at her health club. "I love it, but between getting there, dressing, and showering, I'm always pressed for time," she told John. "How do you do it?"

John smiled and pointed at his walking shoes. "These are my secret weapon," he told her.

Workout Adviser: The Social Aspect of Exercise

If you can find a group of people to exercise with, at least part of the time, you'll discover that workout partners are fantastic aerobic aids. A brisk walk with a friend, while you talk about baseball or the news of the world, flies by with incredible speed. Exercise partners also make it harder to find excuses for ducking a scheduled workout and easier to find reasons for doing them. Look for an office mate who likes to take a healthy stroll from time to time, or recruit friends and family members for a trip to the pool or a spin on your bicycle.

Cycling is an especially social sport, since cyclists can take turns leading the way and breaking up the air resistance for the other cyclists. There's a whole ritual involved, as each rider takes his turn at the front of the pack, then retreats to the end of the line when his turn is done.

Clubs for cycling, walking, running, and swimming exist in almost every medium-sized metropolitan area in the country and in a lot of less-populated regions as well. These clubs can be a great source of workout partners, and they often sponsor instructional classes as well.

You can begin your search for fellow exercisers by calling your local parks and recreation department, or the YMCA. You can also look in the Yellow Pages, under "Athletic Organizations." If you still come up empty, stop in a local athletic shoe store or bike shop— they'll be able to fill you in on what's going on in your town.

If you do hook up with a club, you may even decide to participate in some formal group workouts. Many walking clubs hold group walks, for example. During winter in the northern regions, walking groups will take over shopping malls and sports arenas in the off-hours, turning them into giant, room-temperature gyms.

Lap swimming, which is usually limited to a 25- or 50-yard pool, is the sport most suited to organized workouts. Many swimmers find they get a better workout when they're supervised by a coach who can keep them motivated by varying the workouts and who can offer technical advice and verbal encouragement. This can be important when you're thrashing along in a crowded pool. Many YMCAs and other swimming centers offer swimming workouts for the general public.

Body Maintenance Manual: Keeping Your Back Pain-free

Nothing will kill your exercise plans faster than a bad back. Whether it's a shooting pain, a dull ache, or a wrenching spasm, back pain can quickly turn an active person into a crippled invalid.

Persistent back aches are a huge and expensive health problem. Almost everyone in the United States will have back pain at some time in their lives, at an annual cost to Americans of nearly *$100 billion* dollars—around $20 billion for treating the pain and an estimated $80 billion in lost wages and productivity.

To make matters worse, no one has been able to explain exactly why back pain happens or to come up with a surefire, permanent cure. That's because doctors are still unclear about how our backs work. Unlike other limbs, which move in defined ways, the back has dozens of muscles that let it move in virtually any direction, while supporting huge loads. Your back muscles are the strongest in your body, exerting a force as much as two or three times your body weight in some places along your spine. But if their balance is thrown off, even these ultrastrong muscles can get strained and go into spasm. When that happens, watch out—because the strength is suddenly pulling in a wrong and painful direction.

Doctors now agree that as much as 90 percent of back pain is caused when your back muscles become fatigued and give out. New studies with MRI imaging machines have shown that those old scapegoats called "slipped disks," or vertebrae that are out of alignment, actually have very little connection with back pain. The once-popular spinal operations to fix these bulging discs are now given to less than 1 percent of all back patients.

Since the real culprits are overworked muscles, modern back treatments now begin with a checkup by an orthopedist or another doctor trained in back care and usually progress to some kind of physical therapy program to stretch and strengthen key areas, especially in the lower back itself. Aerobic exercise is often prescribed, too. (Bed rest is another idea that's been retired. Doctors now recommend no more than two days' bed rest for a bad back. More downtime than that will only weaken your muscles further.) Chiropractic treatment has also shown good short-term results as far as relieving immediate pain is concerned. But no manipulation, however artfully done, can make a weak muscle strong. The best chiropractors now usually prescribe exercises for their patients, in addition to hands-on treatment. The goal should be a permanent cure, not weekly treatments that continue indefinitely.

Besides doing special exercises, you can take the following precautions to keep your back healthy and on line:

- Wear shoes with low heels (one inch or less). A raised heel shifts your center of gravity backward, putting additional strain on your back muscles.

- When you lift a heavy object, get as close to it as you can, and lift by first going into a balanced squatting position, then straightening your legs, keeping your back and abdominal muscles tensed. Never lift a heavy load higher than your waist (this puts a huge strain on your back muscles), and never twist to the side while lifting something.

- If you're riding in a car or sitting at a desk, take a break every 30 minutes to stand up, stretch, and walk around for a few minutes. Your body is made for movement, which naturally lubricates your joints: Sitting still for long periods of time reduces this lubrication; that's why you feel stiff after being cramped in one position for a long time.

- When you're sitting for long hours at a desk, it's absolutely essential to have a chair that's fitted exactly to your body measurements. "Making sure their employees have well-made, adjustable chairs at the workplace is one of the most important investments a company will ever make," says Marjorie Koutsandreas, a physical therapist who runs a Maryland-based consulting firm. She counsels large corporations on office design and employee fitness.

"Any office chair should have an adjustable back rest, that you can position so it supports the lumbar curve in the small of your back," Koutsandreas says. If it doesn't, you can go to a medical supply store and buy a lumbar roll (a pillow that fits into the small of your back).

The chair should also have an adjustable seat, so you can pick just the right height to keep your spine stretched and comfortable. If your chair is adjusted correctly, your feet should be flat on the floor as you sit upright, and your hips and thighs should form a right angle.

While most cases of back pain clear up on their own in a week or so, you're risking another episode if you don't take some steps to strengthen your back and trunk muscles. If your back is fine now, the following six exercises can help keep it that way.

Six Back-building Exercises

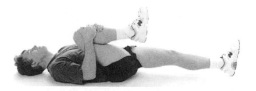

1. SLING STRETCH. If you do one exercise for your back, this should be the one. It gently stretches the muscles of your lower back, bringing healing blood to the area. Done repeatedly, it will strengthen your lower back and lower abdomen.

Lie on your back with your legs straight. Use both hands to pull one knee toward your chest with both hands, until the knee can move no further. Breathe in deeply then exhale, relax, and pull your knee closely to your chest again. Return to starting position. Repeat three to five times with each leg.

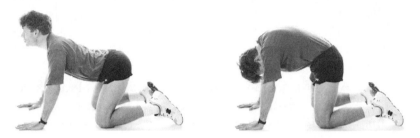

2. MAD CAT STRETCH. This stretch is good for overall trunk flexibility. It makes a good warmup for tennis, basketball, and other sports.

On a rug or some other padded surface, get on your hands and knees and breathe slowly, concentrating on holding your back level. Next, exhale slowly while you contract your stomach muscles and curve your back upward like a dome. Breathe in and return to level position. Then exhale slowly again, and this time arch your back downward, like a suspension bridge.

Do three to five repetitions.

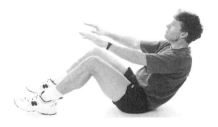

3. SIT-DOWN This "reverse sit-up" exercise works the abdominal muscles more effectively than ordinary curls or sit-ups, according to top back doctors.

Sit on the floor with both knees bent and your feet flat on the floor. Extend your arms out in front of you. Contract your stomach muscles so the bottom of your pelvis tilts up slightly and your lower back flattens out. Holding this position, slowly curl your trunk down almost to the floor, then return to starting position.

Do five to ten repetitions.

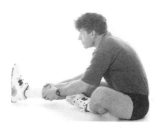

4. HAMSTRING STRETCH (SECOND VERSION)   Sit on the floor with one leg bent so the sole of the foot rests against the inside of your other leg. Gently curl down toward the knee of your straightened leg. When you feel a mild, pleasant tension, stop and hold the stretch, breathing deeply and slowly.

Repeat three times on each leg.

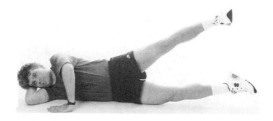

5. LATERAL LIFT.   This exercise strengthens the hips and trunk muscles used in sideways movement. It's a great drill for sports that rely on lateral movement.

Lie on your side with your legs straight. Rest your head on one arm and use your top arm to balance with. Raise both legs off the ground a few inches and hold them there; then raise and lower your upper leg in a slow scissors movement.

Repeat 10 times on each side.

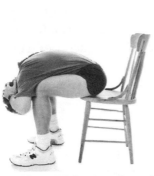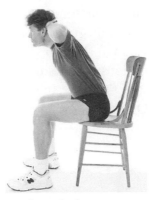

6. BACK LIFT.   This exercise will isolate and work the extensor muscles in your lower back. Weak back extensors are a leading cause of back pain.

Sit on the edge of a chair, bench, or bed, with your feet flat on the floor. Clasp your hands behind your head, and then bend forward at the waist as far as you can. Next, slowly lift your head and trunk upward, until your back is at a 45° angle to the floor. Do 10 repetitions.

Three Exercises to Ease the Pain

When acute pain strikes, a health professional is your best hope. But you might also consider the following three exercises, which are designed to relieve acute pain and keep it from returning.

These exercises come from the McKenzie school of back therapy. This approach is named after its founder, a physical therapist named Robin McKenzie, who developed his methods in his home country of New Zealand. The McKenzie program has now spread all over the world. Its exercises use very gentle movement; repeating them often (six or more times a day) is the secret to their success. These three are meant to be done as a progression. Get comfortable with the first exercise before moving to the second and third.

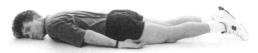

1. LYING FACE DOWN.   Lie face down with your arms beside your body and your head turned to one side. Take a few deep breaths, and then relax *completely,* holding this position for five minutes.

Do this exercise six to eight times a day and at the start of every exercise session.

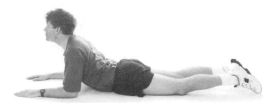

2. LYING EXTENSION.   Lying face down, place your forearms flat on the floor in front of you, so that your elbows are directly under your shoulders. Lean comfortably on your forearms, take a few deep breaths, relax *completely,* and hold this position for five minutes.

Do this exercise six to eight times a day and at the start of every exercise session.

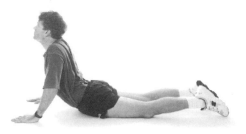

3. ACTIVE EXTENSION.   Lie face down with your palms beneath your shoulders, as if you were about to do a push-up. Straighten your elbows and gently push the top half of your body up as far as pain permits. Keep your pelvis, hips, and legs *completely relaxed* as you do this, and let your lower back sag down. Hold this position for a couple of seconds, then lower yourself back to the floor. Repeat ten times, trying to push your upper body a little higher each time. Do this exercise six to eight times a day.

WEEK EIGHT

TWO 30-MINUTE WORKOUTS
TWO 45-MINUTE WORKOUTS
ONE 60-MINUTE WORKOUT
(TWO STRENGTH WORKOUTS)

Total aerobic time: 3:30 (210 minutes)

Total calories burned: 1260 calories if you weigh 165 lbs.; 1470 calories, 190 lbs.; 1680 calories, 220 lbs.

WEEKLY CHECKLIST

☐ Did I do at least 30 minutes of aerobic activity five times this week?

☐ Did I get in one long aerobic workout?

☐ Did I make healthy choices in what I did and ate?

DAY	50	51	52
WORKOUT:			
COMMENTS:			
RESTING HR:			

WEEK EIGHT

GOAL: To complete your second full month of regular aerobic exercise, maintaining your full load of three-and-a-half hours of aerobic training.

WEEKLY REPORT: Steady improvements should continue, with all aerobic systems in high gear at this point. Look for small but lasting drops in weight (even a fraction of a pound is good—remember, you haven't been dieting!) and continued small reductions in fat levels.

The Workout Adviser this week is about advanced weight lifting, for men who'd like to add a few additional exercises to their strength training program. John Jones has started lifting weights only in the past two weeks—spending a few minutes once a week on the Nautilus equipment at the club where he plays racketball, doing one set apiece on the leg press, leg curl, chest press, and lat pull-down machines. He is not an enthusiastic weight lifter, but his doctor convinced him that strength training even once a week

53	54	55	56

would help him raise his HDL cholesterol levels and help shrink his love handles.

It's too early to see any results from this light strength-training program, but the lifting sessions leave John feeling surprisingly energetic and light on his feet. And the fact that the weight lifting takes so little time—less than 10 minutes, really—is a big plus for our time-pressured hero. The key to efficient exercise, he's beginning to realize, is knowing what you want to do and then doing it, with no dawdling. John calls this "focussing." His wife calls it "rearranging your priorities."

Workout Adviser: Staying Motivated

Remember those college classes where the professor would announce at the beginning that "half of you won't make it to the end of this course"? The same is true of people who start a new exercise program: Research shows that about half of them quit inside 12 months.

How can you avoid being one of these exercise dropouts? Proceeding slowly and carefully is a good start. Another way is to educate yourself about the positive changes happening in your body and then to keep an eye out for signs of improvement.

One sign is increased muscle tone. Even if you haven't lost any pounds in the first two months of your program, you'll still be adding to your muscle mass (which weighs more than fat), and you should see a noticeable increase in muscle size and tone by the end of the second month.

Another indication of progress is reduced levels of body fat. You can observe this by doing an informal "skinfold" test on yourself (described in Appendix G). Watch for small improvements; it means you're moving in the right direction.

The best way to measure your increased aerobic fitness is to take your resting heart rate once a day. Try to take it at the same time every day—when you wake up in the morning, for example, or before you go to bed at night. Over your first three months of exercise, your heart rate should go down steadily, lowering by at least a few beats per minute as your heart begins to pump more and more blood with each contraction. (If your resting heart rate is abnormally high, on the other hand, it could be a sign that you're ill or overtraining.)

Another secret to a successful exercise program is to be clear on what your goals are and why you're pursuing them. Remind yourself frequently that you're giving your body the daily activity it was born for and that you will be healthier for it. Reward yourself for your good habits, and reward your body, too—with a massage, or a hot bath, or a day relaxing at the beach.

Finally, it's important that your family and friends support you in your new life-style. Tell them about your goals, and encourage them to help you meet those goals. If someone expresses impatience with you for taking time out to do your daily exercise, explain why you're doing it, and encourage him or her to join you. With a little luck, you could start a new trend!

Body Maintenance Manual: Advanced Strength Training

A routine of several balanced strength training exercises, done twice a week, will produce steady gains in strength from week to week. Once you get into this routine, however, you may want to expand your program to work more muscle groups or build up your strength faster.

One way to get stronger faster is to add a third strength workout each week. Studies have shown that you can boost your strength gains by 33 percent if you add this extra session. (Always leave one full rest day between strength workouts.)

Another way to further improve your overall strength—especially in your upper body—is to add a few more weight-lifting exercises to the four described in Week Three. If you're ready and willing to spend several extra minutes on each strength training session, Wayne Westcott, strength training consultant for the YMCA, recommends adding the following four weight-lifting exercises to your program. These lifts, together with the four exercises you're already doing, make up what Westcott and others call the "Big 8," addressing all the major muscle groups of the body.

KEEPING YOURSELF COVERED

What's the best way to make sure you stick to your exercise plans? In a study at Michigan State University, the use of multiple incentives, combined with a lot of social support and peer pressure worked best.

Here's how the MSU plan worked: Exercisers drew up a "contract" in which they agreed to exercise for 30 minutes, four times a week, for the next six months—at the same time wagering $40 that they would stick to the contract. They then divided into teams. Anyone who skipped a workout forfeited half his wager and prevented his team from collecting money from other teams for that week. Each exerciser was also required to have someone else "witness" each workout and confirm that it had been completed.

"We weren't really trying to check for liars," explained one of the study's designers. "It was just a way to give the exercisers another layer of social support."

The bottom line is that all this peer pressure worked: A phenomenal 97 percent of the exercisers fulfilled their contract.

You can follow a similar approach on your own. First, make a specific contract about how often you plan to exercise (the Fit Again program is a good start). Next, enlist the support of family and friends: Tell them about your commitment, and ask them to keep tabs on how you're doing. Finally, include rewards for yourself for doing well (like a vacation, or a purchase you've been wanting to make), and punishments (such as household chores) if you fall off the exercise wagon.

Exercise 1: Dumbbell Biceps Curl (or Multi-biceps Machine)

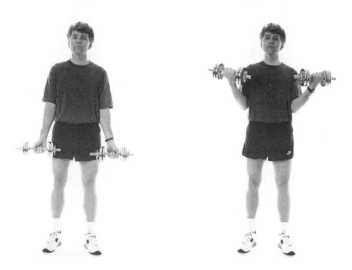

Stand comfortably with your feet slightly apart, and hold both dumbbells down at your side, with your arms fully extended. Keeping your head up and your back straight, slowly curl both dumbbells to your shoulders, counting "one one thousand, two one thousand," and so on. Then slowly lower the dumbbells to starting position, maintaining this same "head up, back straight" posture.

Exercise 2: Dumbbell Triceps Extension (or Multi-triceps Machine)

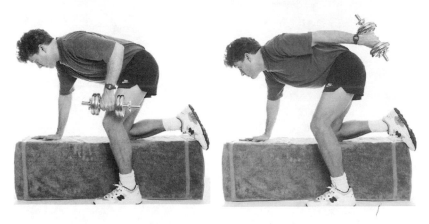

Holding a dumbbell in your left hand, place your free right hand on a bench, and rest your right knee on the bench so that your lower leg is supported. Hold the dumbbell with your palm facing in toward you, and bend your left arm slightly, bringing the weight to rest beside your hip. Without moving your shoulder or upper arm, straighten your lower arm behind you. Then slowly return to starting position. (Think of your elbow as a hinge, opening and closing.) Repeat 8 to 12 times with each arm.

Exercise 3: Dumbbell Shoulder Press (or Overhead Press Machine)

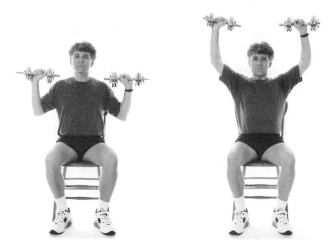

Sit on a bench or chair, with your feet flat on the floor, and hold both dumbbells at shoulder level, your palms facing forward and your elbows pointing downward. Then squeeze your shoulder blades together, and slowly press the weights upward until your arms are straight but not locked. Return slowly to starting position. (The movement should be very controlled—don't use your momentum to help you.) Repeat 8 to 12 times.

Exercise 4: Dumbbell Deltoid Raise (or Lateral Raise Machine)

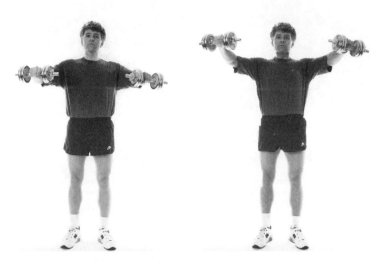

Holding both dumbbells, stand upright with your arms at your sides and your elbows bent at a right angle, palms facing down. Keeping your arms in this position, slowly raise them until your upper arms are horizontal (parallel to the ground). Then slowly lower your arms to starting position, maintaining this same arm position.

BREAKING THROUGH A "PLATEAU"

There may be times in your strength training when you feel "stuck" at a certain weight level and aren't improving as much as you'd like. This is known as a plateau, and it happens to everyone. To break through a plateau, first review the strength training tips in Week Three to be sure you're doing your lifting correctly. Next, begin varying your workouts a little: Try a heavier weight and do fewer repetitions, or a lighter weight and more repetitions. Each approach will stimulate muscle fibers a little differently. Try taking an extra rest day between workouts as well, or switching from dumbbells to a weight machine (or vice versa).

If you're really serious about making a strength breakthrough, you can also try a couple of techniques used by professional athletes to push their muscles beyond what they're used to doing.

Breakdown training involves lifting a weight until you're too tired to do another repetition (this is called "momentary muscle failure"), then *immediately* shifting to a slightly lower weight by having a lighter dumbbell on hand, or moving the key down a couple of notches if you're using a weight machine. For example, if you're bench pressing 120 pounds and your arms give out after the tenth repetition, quickly set the weight machine to 100 pounds and try to lift the weight two or three times more (you can then reduce the weight again, if you want). Each time you shift down, you should reduce the weight by about 15 percent.

Assisted training requires a training partner. It's similar to breakdown training: When you reach the point of "momentary failure" in a given exercise, your partner will grasp the bar you're holding and use his or her muscle power to help you squeeze out a few more repetitions.

"To keep improving," says Westcott, "it's important to experiment with all the different variables in your strength program—the number of repetitions, the type of lifts you're doing, and your recovery period—to see what works best for you. Strength plateaus are overcome not by overtraining but by training more intelligently."

WEEK NINE

TWO 30-MINUTE WORKOUTS

TWO 45-MINUTE WORKOUTS

ONE 60-MINUTE WORKOUT

(TWO TO THREE STRENGTH WORKOUTS)

❖ ❖ ❖

Total aerobic time: 3:30† (210 minutes†)

Total calories burned: 1260 calories if you weigh 165 lbs.; 1470 calories, 190 lbs.; 1680 calories, 220 lbs.

WEEKLY CHECKLIST

☐ Did I do at least 30 minutes of aerobic activity five times this week?

☐ Did I get in one long aerobic workout?

☐ Did I make healthy choices in what I did and ate?

DAY	57	58	59
WORKOUT:			
COMMENTS:			
RESTING HR:			

WEEK NINE

GOAL: To continue making sharp improvements in aerobic fitness, as your body finishes adapting to your full aerobic training load of three-and-a-half hours per week.

WEEKLY REPORT: This is the start of your third month in training. Don't expect your aerobic (slow-twitch) muscle fibers to get much bigger from here on. (If you're lifting weights, your fast-twitch fibers will continue to grow.) But with aerobic power, chemistry counts more than size: This month you can expect to see the biggest gains in endurance of all, as your muscles continue to adjust to a full 200-plus minutes of weekly exercise.

From here on in, you can expand your long workouts up to two hours. That's when the glycogen in your muscles starts to get seriously depleted; it's the point marathoners refer to as "the wall."

You can also begin experimenting with different paces. By speeding and slowing down slightly (while maintaining a comfortable, steady pace), you can work different motor units in your muscles and get a more well-rounded workout. One way to do this, and push yourself a bit at the same time, is interval training, discussed in this week's Workout Adviser.

60	61	62	63

Our man in the middle, John Jones, has naturally gravitated to a varied-pace menu. His walks tend to be leisurely, while he puts in a fairly hard effort on his weekend bike rides. His weekly racketball matches, on the other hand, feature a mix of aerobic action and a lot of short, sprinting movements, which leave him huffing and puffing.

These sprints aren't doing much for his cardiovascular health, but they are providing John's muscles with a different type of workout: an anaerobic workout that develops fast twitch muscle fibers the same way strength training does.

Some occasional anaerobic exercise or fast interval training will help give your muscles an extra chemical edge and a little better tone, and it will also prepare you better for fast-paced sports than aerobics alone will.

Workout Adviser: Interval Training

Interval training is one of the most powerful workout tools ever invented and, in one form or another, is used by virtually every top athlete. In a nutshell, interval training means alternating short bursts (30 to 120 seconds long) of fast walking, cycling, swimming, or running, with stretches of slower effort, which give you a chance to rest and recover before picking up the pace again. These recovery intervals are what gave interval training its name.

This technique allows you to exercise much more intensely than you would if you simply stuck to one pace. For example, you probably couldn't walk 1 mile in 10 minutes. But you *could* walk 1 minute at that pace, covering a tenth of a mile. If you put in 10 fast bursts during a 30-minute walk, with an easier 2-minute recovery in between them, you'll be teaching your body to hold that faster pace without tiring. Along the way, you'll develop more aerobic capacity and burn a few additional calories—and you'll probably find that your workout is more entertaining and exhilarating, too.

Here are some guidelines for planning your own interval workouts:

- Begin with short sections of faster walking or cycling, 20 to 30 seconds long. As you get more experienced, choose any length from 30 seconds to 2 minutes. If you don't have a watch, choose a landmark 100 to 200 yards away and hold your speed until you reach it.

■ Try to keep your form smooth and your pace consistent throughout your fast segments.

■ Your recovery interval should be at least twice as long as your fast segments.

■ Never do two consecutive days of interval training—your body will need time to recover.

■ Don't interval train as part of your weekly "long" workout.

Sample Interval Workout (Walking)

15 minutes moderate-to-brisk walking

21 minutes interval training: 1 minute fast walking, followed by 2 minutes easy walking (repeat 7×)

10 minutes easy-to-moderate walking

Total time: 46 minutes

"Fast" walking time: 7 minutes

Body Maintenance Manual: Defusing Stress

Learning to recognize and deal with stress is as important to your health and well-being as good exercise and nutrition habits are. Stress has many causes, both physical and emotional. But how you *react* to stress is a critical part of the equation.

Your breathing pattern is especially important. Under stress, most people have a tendency to tighten the muscles in their ribs and abdomen, causing their breathing to quicken. Fast breathing causes you to "blow off" too much carbon dioxide, producing a CO_2 deficit in your bloodstream. This triggers immediate chemical changes in your body, cutting oxygen flow to your brain and stimulating your sympathetic ("fight or flight") nervous system, which in turn raises your heart rate and creates an anxious, "wired" feeling.

Over time, rushed breathing or hyperventilation can become

an unnoticed habit. (One subtle sign is frequent sighing or gulping for air.) Chronic overbreathing has been linked to panic attacks and other anxiety disorders. In fact, most garden-variety anxiety, or incessant worrying, is probably your brain's reaction to low carbon dioxide levels. Not only is anxiety distracting, but it's also bad for your health. High levels of anxiety are linked to higher rates of heart disease and may weaken the immune system as well.

Can you cure worry by breathing more slowly? Some psychiatrists think so. Doctors often refer psychotherapy patients to Barbara Wiegand, a New York City breathing therapist, who will work with them to overcome irrational fears by retraining their breathing muscles.

This retraining is a calm, relaxed, slow process since being tense and rushed is what started your overbreathing in the first place. "Everything should be easy," says Wiegand. The goal is to learn how to relax your chest, rib, and shoulder muscles. Wiegand also stresses developing the habit of breathing through your nostrils instead of your mouth. "Nostril breathing is often a revelation to people with bad breathing habits," she notes.

Once you learn and practice a relaxed, easy breathing movement—supplying no more or less air than you actually need—you'll experience a sense of calm, even when your environment may be the opposite. If you practice the following exercises your problems won't disappear, but you'll feel more relaxed and think more clearly, which is probably all you need.

Exercise 1: To Relieve Anxiety

The following "breath retraining" exercise is used by New York City breathing therapist Barbara Wiegand to teach anxiety-prone people how to retool their breathing. Her approach stresses breathing through the nostrils and completely relaxing with each exhalation.

The hardest part, she says, is being patient with the flow of air into your lungs. Because it takes longer for the air flow to reach your lungs, breathing through your nose can feel uncomfortable at first.

Sit in a comfortable position, or lie on your back with your upper body propped up on pillows, at about a 30° angle. (You can also lean all the way back in a reclining chair.)

Focus your complete attention on your nostrils and gently inhale, concentrating on feeling the flow of air through your nose. Next, gently exhale and, at the same time, choose one muscle group (such as your shoulders, arms, or legs) and concentrate on relaxing those muscles as completely as you can. Think of "letting go," making every movement as easy as you can.

Once you've exhaled fully, repeat the process by breathing again. Continue this for 8 to 10 minutes.

To help yourself breathe correctly, you can place a good-sized book, like the telephone directory, on your abdomen. Don't try to move the book as your breathe. Simply *observe* the book rising and falling with each breath.

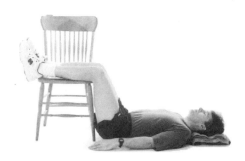

Exercise 2: Muscle Relaxer

This exercise is adapted from Dr. Mary Schatz's book *Back Care Basics* (Rodmell Press). It will promote a relaxed body and calm state of mind, and it is especially helpful if you have tight or sore back muscles.

Lie on your back with your lower legs raised up on the seat of a chair. If you like, put a rolled-up towel under your neck for added support.

Close your eyes and inhale naturally through your nose. Then relax and exhale naturally, also through your nose.

As you finish exhaling, pause *without holding your breath* and silently count "one thousand one, one thousand two," and so on, allowing your exhalation to come to a natural, unforced conclusion.

Repeat for several minutes, keeping your eyes closed and letting your chest and abdomen expand with each in breath.

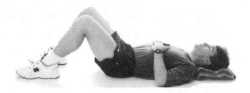

Exercise 3: A Quick Mental Tune-up

The following exercise is really a mini-meditation. It should give you an immediate feeling of physical and mental tranquility.

Sit, or lie on your back, relax, and close your eyes. Begin breathing easily, and simply listen to the sound of your breath going in and out. If your attention drifts away from the sound, gently guide your thoughts back to it. Continue for several minutes. For added relaxation, pick a word—it could be *calm,* or *peace,* or any other word you prefer—and repeat that word silently to yourself each time you exhale.

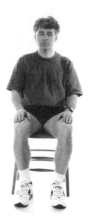

Exercise 4: Rocking Meditation

This exercise is a favorite of Dr. Jonathan Smith, director of the School of Psychology and the Stress Institute at Roosevelt University in Chicago, and author of *Creative Stress Management* (Prentice-Hall).

As you're sitting or standing, close your eyes and begin rocking very gently. Don't worry about your breathing: Just quietly pay attention to the rocking movement of your body.

Next, let the rocking movement become smaller and smaller, until it's so imperceptible that a person sitting next to you would barely notice the motion. Continue attending to this gentle rocking for several minutes. If your mind wanders, that's okay—just gently return to attending to the rocking motion. (You may need to do this many times in a single session.)

"I've found more beginners prefer this type of meditation than any other meditation technique," says Smith. "You can use it almost anywhere—at work, or even on a crowded subway car."

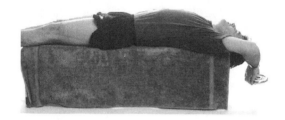

Exercise 5: Breathing Stretch

Holding a light weight in both hands, lie on your back on a bench, a low table, or a bed, so that your neck and arms extend off the end. Keeping your arms parallel, slowly lower the weight back over your head, bending your elbows and inhaling deeply. You'll feel a stretch in your ribs and stomach. Hold the stretch for 10 seconds, then exhale completely, returning to starting position.

WEEK TEN

(DAYS 64–70)

TWO 30-MINUTE WORKOUTS

TWO 45-MINUTE WORKOUTS

ONE 60-MINUTE WORKOUT

(TWO TO THREE STRENGTH WORKOUTS)

Total aerobic time: 3:30† (210 minutes†)

Total calories burned: 1260 calories if you weigh 165 lbs.; 1470 calories, 190 lbs.; 1680 calories, 220 lbs.

WEEKLY CHECKLIST

☐ Did I do at least 30 minutes of aerobic activity five times this week?

☐ Did I get in one long aerobic workout?

☐ Did I make healthy choices in what I did and ate?

DAY	64	65	66
WORKOUT: COMMENTS:			
RESTING HR:			

Week Ten

GOAL: To continue major aerobic improvements, while maintaining a healthy life-style of low-fat eating and some light strength training.

WEEKLY REPORT: You should be starting to feel like a seasoned endurance athlete. If you've been getting your full prescribed exercise, you may well have raised your oxygen-burning capacity 25 percent by now!

In the days of prehistory, getting enough exercise was never a problem; the big issue was getting enough *food* to fuel this movement. Today things are different. The main challenge facing all of us is finding the free time for daily aerobic activity. This gets even tougher when bad weather hits. If you're dressed properly, then cold weather doesn't have to be a problem (which is the topic of this week's Workout Adviser, by the way), but rain, snow, and ice are another story.

Unless you live somewhere like Los Angeles or Phoenix, in

67	68	69	70

order to keep your long-range exercise plans on track, you'll need to develop an emergency fall-back plan for days when bad weather strikes. This could be a piece of indoor exercise equipment, like a NordicTrack or a treadmill, or it could be an indoor walking area, such as a shopping mall or an underground concourse. It doesn't have to be a form of exercise you love—just something you can turn to for your all-important 30 minutes of aerobics when you're snowed in for the weekend, or when the rain pours down for the second day in a row.

John Jones has his own bad-weather solution: After he'd been exercising for several weeks, he dragged a motorized treadmill in from the garage—a birthday gift of two years ago that he'd almost never used. He retrieved it out of curiosity, but after he gave the machine a 10-minute test walk he discovered that walking in his living room was kind of fun.

Now, if rain wipes out his morning walk, John comes home at night and takes a 30-minute walk while he watches the evening news. His improved fitness allows him to pass on his editorial comments to anyone in earshot, which includes most of the house.

Workout Adviser: Dealing With Cold Weather

Many an exercise program has been derailed in the winter months, when darkness comes early and the cold winds start to blow. But really, exercising in cold weather is one of the easiest adjustments you'll ever make. A regular wintertime walk can actually turn the cold into an enjoyable encounter, and also provide a welcome break from being cooped up indoors. If you are one of the millions of men and women who get hit by blue moods in the winter (known as seasonal affective disorder, or S.A.D.), it also provides a chance to expose yourself to some direct sunlight on a daily basis—a treatment that boosts levels of the brain chemical serotonin, reversing the syndrome and elevating your mood.

The secret to successful winter exercise is to dress for it, and winter clothing can be summed up in a word: *synthetics.* The days of wearing cotton or silk next to your skin are long gone. Why? Because these materials quickly get soaked with sweat and then sit next to your skin, creating a wet and clammy environment that's bound to make you uncomfortable sooner or later.

"The microenvironment on the surface of your skin determines how you feel, no matter what the weather is," says Dr. Murray Hamlet, director of research and operations at the Army Research Institute of Environmental Medicine. "If that tiny area between your skin and your first layer of clothing is cold and wet, you'll *feel* cold and wet. If it's warm and dry, you'll feel quite comfortable."

The underwear of choice today is polypropylene, or a similar synthetic material. The beauty of these fabrics is that they wick sweat away from your skin, while retaining their insulating properties. The result: You stay happy, warm, and dry, and cold weather exercise turns into a remarkably pleasant adventure.

Here's a rundown on how to prepare for the winter chill:

- Start taking note of the cold when the mercury hits 40°F or even slightly higher if the weather is misty or if there's a stiff breeze (which will whip away the mini-atmosphere on your skin's surface, creating the so-called wind chill effect).

- Move more slowly in cold weather, and opt for smooth terrain: The cold weather makes the fluid in your joints more viscous, like oil in a car, meaning you won't be as spry as you are on warmer days.

- Dress for maximum comfort: Always begin with a bottom layer of synthetic fabric longjohns, top and bottom. You should find them in stores that sell athletic clothing or camping gear. Look for polypropylene, or a polypropylene-cotton blend, or a similar material.

- On very cold days, wear a middle layer of a thick, light material that will help trap warm air, especially on your upper body. Hamlet recommends a garment made of synthetic fleece (Synchilla and Polar-Tec are two well-known brands).

- For your outer layer, wear a wind-resistant shell, such as a rain suit or a Windbreaker.

- Top off your cold-weather exercise outfit with a knit wool cap, mittens (which circulate warm air among your fingers better than gloves do), and a pair of polypropylene socks inside a pair of wool socks.

- Remember to drink a pint of water before exercising—you'll still be sweating a fair amount despite the cool weather.

- If you're taking a cold-weather walk, try to go with a training partner, or tell someone where you're going, and stick with a familiar route. In the cold, an accident can turn dangerous in a hurry.

Middle layer: A synthetic fleece-type pullover, which is light but bulky, good for trapping a layer of warm air.

Bottom layer: Long underwear, tops and bottoms, made out of lightweight polypropylene (or a similar fabric). This material wicks away sweat from your skin, keeping the skin's surface as dry as toast.

On your head: A knit wool cap.

Outer layer: A nylon shell, such as a Windbreaker or rain suit, to keep breezes from penetrating your protective cocoon. In medium-cold weather, use just the top. As the mercury drops, add nylon bottoms, too.

Also recommended: Wool mittens, rather than gloves— they allow warm air to circulate among your fingers.

Informed exercisers know that layers of synthetic clothing are the secret to staying warm and dry, even when the thermometer dips toward zero.

Body Maintenance Manual: Advanced Balance Drills for Improved Sports Performance

The following group of exercises was developed by John Blievernicht, head of the Sports C.A.R.E. rehabilitation clinic in Chicago.

Blievernicht has taken many athletes through his balance-enhancement program at his Chicago clinic—including several N.B.A. stars. "Whether you're lifting a garbage can, returning a tennis serve, or blocking someone on the football field, balance equals strength and speed," he says. "If you're off-balance, anyone can knock you over, and any shot you try will be more difficult."

Advanced Balance Exercises

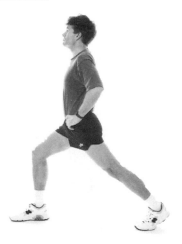

1. LUNGE.   Standing with your feet at shoulder width and your hands on your hips, step forward with one foot and bend your forward leg so that your kneecap is directly over your foot. Hold for 15 seconds. Repeat several times on each leg.

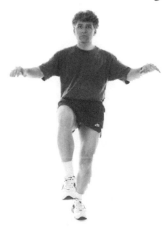

2. ONE-LEGGED SQUAT.   First, practice the one-legged stand until you can do it easily for 15 to 30 seconds on either leg.

Next, stand with your arms relaxed at your sides. Lift one leg off the ground, balancing on the other leg. Slowly bend the leg you're standing on at the hip and knee, keeping your foot pointed straight ahead and your kneecap over your foot. Bend the leg until you feel slightly wobbly, then hold for 15 seconds. Repeat 5 to 10 times on each leg.

Progression: Level one—both eyes open. Level two—one eye closed. Level three—both eyes closed.

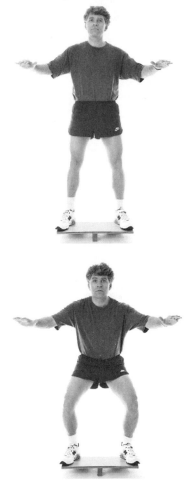

3. BALANCE BOARD.   One of the best ways to wake up the nerves in your legs, feet, and inner ear is to practice standing on an unstable apparatus, like a balance board (basically a flat board with a ridge down the middle—see below for information on where these can be obtained), a mini-trampoline, or even a foam cushion.

First, practice standing tall with good posture on the balance board, trying to hold this for 15 to 30 seconds at a time.

Once this becomes easy, you can progress to a slight squatting movement: Stand balanced on the board, then slowly bend both legs at the knees and hips, until your reach a point where you feel wobbly. Hold for 15 seconds. Repeat several times.

When this is mastered, you can progress to squat repetitions: Stand balanced on the board and slowly bend both legs, then immediately straighten up again. Do 10 to 15 repetitions.

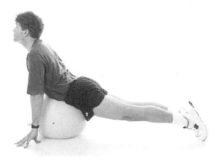

4. BACK EXTENSION ON STABILITY BALL.   Finally, if you're really serious about your balance, Blievernicht recommends investing in a "stability ball," which inflates like a beach ball but has a tough outer skin that can easily bear a person's weight. Doing exercises on the stability ball forces the muscles on both sides of your trunk to work equally. Balance boards (ranging in cost from $25 to $45) and stability balls (at $25) can both be obtained from MF Athletic Company in Cranston, Rhode Island. For mail-order information call 800-556-7464.

This exercise works the muscles of the erector spinae, along the backbone. To do a back extension on the ball, lie with your lower abdomen resting on the top of the ball, with your legs straight and the balls of your feet touching the floor. Leave your arms at your sides (you can touch the floor for added support if you want.) Slowly arch your back upward, and hold for several seconds. Repeat 10 to 15 times.

WEEK ELEVEN

(DAYS 71–77)

Two 30-minute workouts

Two 45-minute workouts

One 60-minute workout

(two to three strength workouts)

❖ ❖ ❖

Total aerobic time: 3:30† (210 minutes†)

Total calories burned: 1260 calories if you weigh 165 lbs.; 1470 calories, 190 lbs.; 1680 calories, 220 lbs.

WEEKLY CHECKLIST

☐ Did I do at least 30 minutes of aerobic activity five times this week?

☐ Did I get in one long aerobic workout?

☐ Did I make healthy choices in what I did and ate?

DAY	71	72	73
WORKOUT:			
COMMENTS:			
RESTING HR:			

WEEK ELEVEN

GOAL: To continue building aerobic capacity by maintaining a schedule of three-and-a-half hours per week with one long workout of an hour or more, and mixing in occasional interval sessions.

WEEKLY REPORT: As your fitness builds, your sped-up metabolism will flush antibodies through your system faster, and it should help you weather minor illnesses better. But being fit doesn't protect you from being infected by colds or flu, especially if other stresses are wearing you down. So remember, if you're feeling rundown or overtired, don't be shy about skipping a few days of exercise. Sometimes your body just needs a rest.

Good fitness also gives only partial protection against hot weather, another natural enemy of the exerciser. Your sweat rate goes up when you're in good shape, giving you some additional cooling effect (the notion that you sweat more when you're out of shape is strictly a myth). But if you plan on exercising in really high temperatures, you need to spend a couple of weeks acclimating once you hit the hot climate. During that time, your sweat rate will practically double.

The other key to heat survival (the topic of this week's Workout Adviser) is to drink water and then drink more water. John

74	75	76	77

Jones carries a quart of the stuff on his bicycle now when he does his hour rides on Saturday and Sunday. By the way, he's now pedalling a brand new $500 twelve-speed bike, a "good work and keep it up" surprise from his wife and kids.

Workout Adviser: Handling the Heat

The biggest danger to any exerciser occurs when the thermometer starts to creep above 80°. Our bodies are equipped to deal with heat, but only up to a point, and only after an adjustment period lasting about two weeks.

If you don't take the proper precautions, hot weather can quickly cut short your daily walk or other aerobic activity. The main threat is dehydration: When you sweat, your three million sweat glands suck microscopic amounts of liquid out of your bloodstream. As you become more dehydrated, your blood plasma literally becomes thicker, making it harder to push blood through the narrow capillaries to your muscles. If you lose even 5 percent of your body weight in perspiration, your muscles' performance will start to suffer.

Without enough water in your system, heat exhaustion can occur within 30 minutes. The most typical sign is a throbbing headache; other symptoms are tingling sensations in your arms or back, chills, or gooseflesh—all signs that your thermoregulatory system isn't working right. Most victims of heat exhaustion recover quickly after they stop exercising and drink enough water to rehydrate.

Sunstroke, a more serious condition, requires more drastic action. This medical emergency comes on very fast, sometimes in just a few minutes. It's caused by strenuous effort in very hot weather— for example, running three miles in the heat of the afternoon. Putting out so many calories, your body overheats faster than sweat can cool you, to the point where your entire temperature control system shuts down. The symptoms are red, dry skin, dizziness, and sometimes fainting. The usual treatment is to cool the patient in a tub of ice water.

The number one rule of hot-weather exercise: Keep everything *easy* in the heat—no hard or long efforts allowed. Save it for a cooler day!

Here are some other ways to have it made in the shade, even on the hottest of days.

■ Allow yourself two weeks to fully adjust to a hot climate by exercising for a short period of time each day in the full heat. Your body will adapt to the new environment by raising the amount of liquid in your blood plasma by up to 20 percent in just three to five days, giving you a larger reservoir to draw on when you perspire and a cushion against dehydration. Also your skin blood flow will gradually decline and your sweat output will go up. After two weeks in a desert climate you'll be perspiring about 30 percent more liquid than before you were acclimatized.

■ Exercise in the early morning or evening whenever possible. This is when temperatures are coolest and also when ground ozone (a dangerous by-product of car exhaust) is at its lowest.

■ Drink, drink, drink. Take in as much water as you can during the day, and make a point of drinking a pint to a quart of non-carbonated liquid 15 minutes before your workout. And drink as often during the workout as you feel you need to. Most heat experts agree that water is the beverage of choice, although electrolyte-laced sports drinks may give you an edge in exercise that lasts more than an hour. Any fruit juice you drink should be diluted with water to prevent stomach upset.

   If you've been sweating heavily, or exercising in a hot breeze, be sure to drink water even when you don't feel especially thirsty: Your thirst mechanism tends to lag behind when you're dehydrating quickly.

■ Check the color of your urine to see how well-hydrated your body is. Light yellow is ideal; dark yellow means you need to drink a few glasses of water.

■ Don't be fooled into thinking you're sweating less in a hot, dry climate, just because your clothes aren't drenched. You'll actually sweat 5 to 10 percent *more* in a dry climate, but your perspiration evaporates much more quickly.

■ Don't expect much from ducking under a lawn sprinkler: Studies by the U.S. Army showed that even a full 30-second shower of cool water had virtually no effect on the body temperature of overheated soldiers.

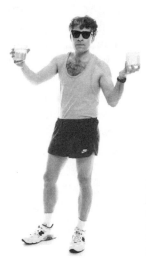

In hot weather, it's important to drink *more* than you think you need, to prevent dehydration and possible heat exhaustion. On a hot day, experts recommend drinking a full quart of water 15 minutes before you head out the door to exercise.

Body Maintenance Manual: Cycling Tips

Much of the world uses the bicycle as a main form of transportation. In the United States, bikes have a long way to go before they supplant our car culture—but cycling *has* taken a huge leap in popularity over the last 10 years. At least 20 million adult Americans now cycle regularly for fitness.

Major advances in bike technology have helped to spur this cycling boom. Today's bikes are lighter, better made, and more user-friendly than ever before. But the most important innovation has been the development of the mountain bike, and its cousin, the hybrid bike.

Mountain bikes combine the high-tech gears and brakes of the traditional road bicycle with a structure that looks like the old "clunker" bicycles you probably learned to ride on: The handlebars are straight, not curved—allowing you to pedal without hunching over—and the tires are fat, with tough, treated rubber. The frame is heavier than a road bike, and the seat is broader and flatter. Some models even have shock-absorbers built in.

These sturdy, upright bikes were first designed by people who enjoyed riding on steep, twisty mountain paths and wanted a bike that could stand up to the punishment. But the bikes have caught on with the general public in a big way, since they fulfill a common wish: To have a multi-gear bike that's as easy and comfortable to ride as the one-speed bikes we all rode on as kids. Today, sales of mountain bikes and hybrids (slimmed-down versions that are a cross between a mountain and a touring bike) account for half of the 10 million new bicycles purchased each year in the United States.

Buying a bike is the first step in starting a cycling program. The next step is to learn the basics of safe, effective cycling, and find a lightly trafficked neighborhood where you can put your skills into action.

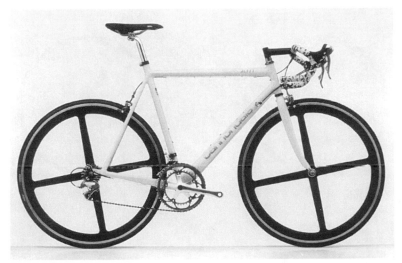

Road bike

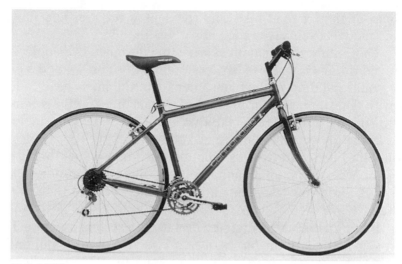

Hybrid bike

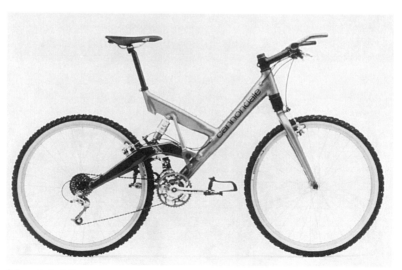

Mountain bike

The Cyclist's Guide

- If you want a well-made bike that will give you years of use, be ready to spend about $400. If you pay less, you're running the risk of buying a less solidly built bike that will break down under heavy use or start to operate imperfectly.

   When buying a bike, go to an established bike store staffed by experienced cyclists, who can steer you to a model suited to your needs and your wallet.

- An expert bike shop will also make sure that the frame size of your bike is fitted to your body size and that the seat and handlebars are carefully adjusted as well—otherwise you'll end up with an aching back or neck. As a general rule, the seat is at the correct height if your leg is fully extended at the bottom of the pedalling motion.

- Before you head out for an extended ride, spend a day or two acquainting yourself with your bike. Find a flat, quiet street or an empty parking lot, and practice switching gears as you ride, until the process starts to feel natural and you can change gears without interrupting your pedalling rhythm. You'll notice that it's much easier to pedal in the lower gears, but you'll cover less ground with each pedal stroke. Higher gears let you cover ground faster, and they also require more leg power on each stroke.

   Another trick that may take some practice is braking with both hands simultaneously. If you pull on just the front-wheel brake, you could find yourself flying over the handlebars, since the back of your bike will still be moving forward.

   Finally, you should also practice turning to look quickly over your shoulder as you ride. This is an all-important safety maneuver whenever you're around automobiles or other cyclists.

- Once you feel secure handling your bicycle, pick a short loop and ride it a few times, working on your pedalling cadence. This term refers to how fast you turn the pedals as you ride. The key to cycling for 30 minutes or more is to maintain a high cadence, which prevents you from overtaxing your muscles.

The ideal cadence is between 80 and 90 complete pedal revolutions per minute. This means pumping both legs in less than a second, a tempo that's *faster* than a normal walking stride. Beginning cyclists tend to ride at a slower cadence of around 60 revolutions per minute, which may feel easier over the short haul but requires more leg strength. This extra burden will tire your legs out after just a few miles.

Do your best to adopt the habit of pedalling at a fast cadence as you ride. To figure out your cadence, use your watch to count how many pedal revolutions you make in 30 seconds, and multiply by 2. To pick up your cadence, simply switch to a slightly lower gear: You'll find your pedalling tempo will increase automatically as the pedalling becomes easier.

■ After you've gotten the basics down, you'll be ready for a real ride. Follow a traffic-free route of three or four miles, using elapsed time as your guide. As your fitness improves, you'll feel a natural urge to lengthen your rides. Because bicycles are such efficient machines, they let you work at a relatively higher aerobic rate than you can achieve by walking or running. This means you can cycle easily for long periods of time and burn some serious calories along the way.

THE RULES OF SAFE CYCLING

For thrills without any serious spills, always follow these rules of bike safety:

1. Before you head out, be sure that your tires are properly inflated and that your brakes and gearshift are working correctly.
2. If you ride at night, wear reflective clothing and use a bike light.
3. Avoid slippery surfaces such as sand, loose gravel, oil spills, or roads slick from rain or fallen leaves.

4. Always ride on the right side of the road, with traffic.

5. Yield to all cross-traffic.

6. If automobiles or other cyclists are in the vicinity, clearly signal all your movements in advance. Hold your left arm straight out to the side for a left turn, and your right arm out to the side for a right turn. Signal that you're about to stop by pointing your left arm down toward the ground.

7. If you're riding with other cyclists, maintain a single file. Always pass other riders on the left, and call out "on your left" loudly as you do.

8. For the smoothest ride, you should oil the bearings in your wheel hubs often—once a week, if possible. Check with a bike shop to see what oil is best for your bike.

9. Carry identification whenever you ride.

10. *Always* wear a bike helmet when you cycle. Look for a helmet with a Snell or ANSI sticker inside, which shows that it's been crash-tested.

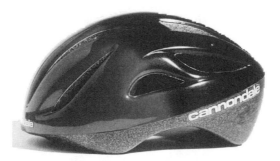

WEEK TWELVE

(DAYS 78–84)

TWO 30-MINUTE WORKOUTS

TWO 45-MINUTE WORKOUTS

ONE 60-MINUTE WORKOUT

(TWO TO THREE STRENGTH WORKOUTS)

Total aerobic time: 3:30† (210 minutes†)

Total calories burned: 1260 calories if you weigh 165 pounds; 1470 calories, 190 l.,; 1680 calories, 220 lbs.

WEEKLY CHECKLIST

☐ Did I do at least 30 minutes of aerobic activity five times this week?

☐ Did I get in one long aerobic workout?

☐ Did I make healthy choices in what I did and ate?

DAY	78	79	80
WORKOUT:			
COMMENTS:			
RESTING HR:			

WEEK TWELVE

GOAL: To complete your sixth week of 200-plus minutes' aerobic training and begin to establish the new, higher plane of fitness that you will continue on after the end of 90 days.

WEEKLY REPORT: Your weekly five-workout routine should be second nature by this twelfth week, and you shouldn't be feeling any muscle tiredness or soreness on the day after your workouts. If you do, you're pushing too hard and should ease up on the pace of your daily aerobics.

But even if you stay within the parameters of safe, smart exercise, your body is bound to feel some wear and tear as those weeks of walking, cycling, or swimming start to add up. This comes with the territory—and so you need to make a special effort to relax, unwind, and untense your muscles whenever you can. One good approach is to stretch your muscles several times a week, following the program outlined in Week Five. Another method is pro-

81	82	83	84

gressive muscle relaxation: Lie down with your eyes closed, and begin tensing and then relaxing various groups of muscles. Begin with the shoulders and arms, and move downward toward your legs.

Massage and whirlpool therapy are also good for tired, overused muscles, but if you don't have a massage therapist or a whirlpool bath handy, try standing in a hot shower for 10 minutes.

Any more aggressive treatments should be cleared with your doctor first. John Jones got his physician's okay for a twice-weekly sauna at his racketball club. His doc doesn't think it does much for him physically one way or the other, but the regular baking makes John feel incredibly relaxed and healthy—a placebo effect that can only help his health and sense of well-being.

Workout Adviser: Water Workouts

If you spend an occasional day at the beach, you've got a ready-made walking course, down and back along the surf. But you can also get an extra workout by walking in knee-deep water. This strengthens the muscles in the front of each hip, which work hard every time you lift your leg to step forward.

You can get a similar effect by walking in the shallow end of a pool. Or you can wear a buoyant vest (available in sporting goods stores) and literally walk across the pool by treading water with your legs. This type of water aerobics is especially valuable for people with sore knees or backs, who may find extended walking to be painful or fatiguing.

There are also water exercises designed for people with arthritis, to relieve the pain and restore free movement in crippled joints. The following four pool exercises were developed by Dvera Berson, author of *Pain-Free Arthritis,* (S & J Books, Brooklyn, N.Y.) who helped cure her own severe arthritis through water exercise. They were developed for arthritis patients, but anyone who tries these exercises will feel more relaxed and limber afterwards.

Four Anti-Arthritis Exercises

1. *Finger strengthener:* Stand in waist-high water, with your arms hanging comfortably at your sides. Holding your hands in the water, flutter each finger on both hands forward and back while moving your thumbs up and down. All fingers should be moving at once, with each finger moving independently of the others. All movements should be slow and gentle, so that you can feel your fingers pushing the water.

2. *Shoulder and upper-back strengthener:* Standing in neck-deep water, slowly cross your arms in front of you at the elbows, then slowly and gently swing them behind you as far they'll comfortably go. Feel your arms pushing the water forward, then back, as you move.

3. *Back, knee, ankle, and wrist relaxer:* Standing in chin-high water, lift your left knee up as high as you can, and at the same time lift your right arm and wrist up and back, as if you were a waiter carrying a tray. Keep your wrists and ankles as relaxed as you can. Next, repeat with your right knee and left arm. As you lift your knee high, you should feel a stretch in your lower back.

4. *Total body conditioner:* Float on your back, with your arms and legs submerged. Slowly raise your left arm and leg a few inches, then lower them again, as you raise your right arm and leg slightly. Repeat indefinitely. With practice, you can learn to propel yourself around the pool using this movement.

Body Maintenance Manual: Swimming Tips

There's a good reason why U.S. Olympic swimmers have dominated the world for decades. America is a swimming country: According to the National Sporting Goods Association, over 70 million Americans take a dip each year. Of this group, about 25 million swim laps regularly to keep in shape—making swimming the second-most-popular fitness activity in the country, after walking.

While competitive swimmers train for hours each day, trying to push their muscles to the limit, you can get plenty of health and fitness benefits from 30 to 60 minutes of steady, enjoyable lap swimming and finish feeling relaxed and rejuvenated. Because you're free of gravity as you swim, there's virtually no impact on your bones, making it ideal for people with arthritis, sore knees, or chronic back pain.

"Young or old, slim or overweight, everyone's equal in the pool," says Jane Katz, Ed.D., aquatics professor at John Jay College of Criminal Justice in New York City and the author of *Swimming for Total Fitness* (Doubleday). "Remember," she adds, "your apparent body weight in chin-deep water is about one-tenth of what you weigh on land."

While your training may not be Olympian, that doesn't mean you can't borrow a few training tips from the top swimmers. Here's some advice on how to get the most out of your pool time:

The Swimmer's Guide

- All lap swimming should be done in a pool that has a supervising trained lifeguard. If you swim at home, do so only when someone else is there.
- Warm up and cool down from your lap swimming with a few water exercises. Katz especially recommends three exercises from her *Water Exercise Techniques Workout* book and video:
- Water walking—in chest-deep water, walk several steps forward, backward, sideways, and diagonally.
- The water punch—stand in shoulder-high water and punch straight out at the water, first with one arm, then with the other.
- The over-arm stretch—in shoulder-high water, hold your hands together and reach up toward the sky, moving your hips side to side slightly as you stretch upward. (This is the same streamlined position you want to hold as you swim.)
- Most fitness swimmers use the crawl, also called freestyle, as their main swimming stroke, employing other strokes for a change of pace. When you're swimming freestyle, concentrate first and foremost on developing a relaxed, rhythmic breath-

ing pattern. Breathe once for every two arm strokes, so that you're breathing on the same side of your body each time. (When you get more proficient, you can try alternate-side breathing.)

If you find yourself panting for breath while you swim, you're probably holding your breath without realizing it, says Katz. Whatever stroke you're using, concentrate on *exhaling fully* through your nose and mouth before you breathe in again.

"Watch for your air bubbles, to be sure you're getting a good exhalation," suggests Katz. "Get to know your own air bubbles, so you feel comfortable with them. They're a sign that you're breathing correctly."

- As you swim the freestyle stroke, always keep your elbow higher than your hand, with your fingers pointing slightly downward. This trick will help you maintain an efficient arm stroke.

- Most of your swimming power comes from your arms. Try to kick your legs just hard enough to keep your legs afloat— "enough just to make the water boil slightly, but no more than that," says Katz.

- Pace yourself as you swim, and don't hesitate to break up your swimming into manageable sections, taking a rest break in between. "A common mistake beginners make is to swim very hard for a few laps, until they're so tired they can't continue," says Katz. "You're better off swimming two laps, resting, then doing two more."

- Wear a tight-fitting, competition-style bathing suit when you're swimming laps. Boxer-style trunks will trap water and increase your drag. To protect your eyes from chlorine, wear goggles that fit tightly over your eyes, so they're seated inside the eye socket (like those made by Speedo).

- When sharing a lane with other swimmers, the rule of thumb is that everyone swims in a counterclockwise direction, keeping as close to the right side of the lane as possible at all times. The idea is to stay out of the way of other swimmers. As Katz says, "Swimming doesn't have to be a contact sport!"

WEEK THIRTEEN

(DAYS 85–91)

TWO 30-MINUTE WORKOUTS

TWO 45-MINUTE WORKOUTS

ONE 60-MINUTE WORKOUT

(TWO TO THREE STRENGTH WORKOUTS)

Total aerobic time: 3:30† (210 minutes†)

Total calories burned: 1260 calories if you weigh 165 lbs.; 1470 calories 190 lbs.; 1680 calories, 220 lbs.

WEEKLY CHECKLIST

☐ Did I do at least 30 minutes of aerobic activity five times this week?

☐ Did I do one long aerobic workout?

☐ Did I make healthy choices in what I did and ate?

DAY	85	86	87
WORKOUT:			
COMMENTS:			
RESTING HR:			

Week Thirteen

GOAL: To successfully finish your thirteenth consecutive week of regular aerobic exercise, and to prepare for what lies ahead after the conclusion of your 90-day program. The aim is to make a transition into a permanent life-style of daily exercise, for maximum health and fitness.

WEEKLY REPORT: Congratulations! You've just had your most profitable quarter-year in recent memory—as far as your body is concerned. Right now, your aerobic capacity is probably close to 33 percent greater than it was when you took that first 15-minute walk, 90 days ago. Your muscles have new tone, your step has a new spring to it, and you've most likely moved down a size in your waistband. But the biggest gains are marked by what others can't see: a lower resting heart rate and a stronger heart; the knowledge and confidence that your body can take you an hour's distance or more without tiring; and the hard-won endurance in your muscles themselves.

88	89	90	91

This feeling of inner fitness is what it's all about. The compliments quickly fade away, as John Jones discovered after a month or so. He's quickly gone from being "the guy who used to work out" to "the guy who works out," and most of his friends and coworkers have accepted the new, slimmer John as a given by now.

This doesn't mean John doesn't have a few tricks left up his sleeve. For one thing, he's been getting more interested in cycling and is toying with the idea of training for a "century"—a 100-mile bike ride. He's even been seen reading a bicycling magazine now and then. His wife and friends are eyeing the trend warily. Will John's somewhat obsessive tendencies find a new outlet? Will this threaten the hours he spends biking with his wife, which they both treasure? Only time (or perhaps a sequel) will tell . . .

Workout Adviser: The Road Ahead (How to Be Your Own Coach)

Well, this is it—90 days, as far as the Fit Again schedule can take you. From here on in, it's up to you to map out your exercise strategy and then put it into action on a consistent basis.

The knowledge you've gained reading this book should help guide you. A half-hour or more of aerobic exercise, five days a week, should remain the cornerstone of your weekly routine. Use your 13-week diary as a model for the future.

It will also help if you remind yourself from time to time why this daily exercise is so good for your health:

- It raises your HDL cholesterol and statistically reduces your risk of a heart attack.
- It keeps your muscles toned and durable, prevents adult diabetes, and will improve your mood and raise your energy level.
- It's the most effective way to permanently lower your level of body fat.
- It will increase your expected life span by two years or more.

For additional motivation to stay consistent, remind yourself that *three to four weeks* of total inactivity are all it takes for muscle enzyme levels to start dropping back down into couch potato country. It's not a bad idea to take a week or two off occasionally—most athletes have periods of down time, when they exercise lightly or not at all. This gives a chance for small aches to mend and for muscle fibers to rest and rebuild. But don't make it an indefinite vacation.

The other important aspect of being your own coach is to listen to your body. If it's sore, treat the ache and reevaluate your exercise technique and equipment to see what might be causing the problem. If a nagging pain persists, don't hesitate to see a health care professional. Your body is your passport to health, and you should take scrupulous care to see that it's always in top condition.

Listening to your body also means staying within yourself when you exercise. Never abruptly increase the length or intensity of your workouts—all changes should be gradual. The same is true if you start a new aerobic activity: Begin with slow, short workouts, because as fit as you may be, your body hasn't had a chance to prepare itself for the stress caused by a new movement pattern.

Finally, being your own coach means giving yourself plenty of credit for taking care of your body and giving it the food and exercise it needs. It's the right thing, and the responsible thing, to do.

Body Maintenance Manual: How HDL Cholesterol Levels Affect Your Health

If your doctor is still giving you one blanket figure for your cholesterol count, he or she is behind the times. The data from the 35-year Framingham (Mass.) Heart Study (the longest ongoing heart survey in the United States) clearly shows that *total cholesterol* in the bloodstream isn't what predicts your chances of a heart attack. The best indicator of risk is your cholesterol ratio, gotten by dividing your total by your "high-density lipoprotein" (HDL) cholesterol—the "good" cholesterol, which is responsible for removing fatty molecules from your bloodstream.

Total cholesterol/HDL cholesterol = Cholesterol ratio

For example, if your total cholesterol is 200 and your HDL count is 50, your cholesterol ratio is 4.

This means that low HDLs are just as bad as high levels of low-density lipoprotein (LDL, or "bad") cholesterol. Experts think that as many as a million Americans with apparently normal total cholesterol readings actually have heart disease because of low HDL cholesterol levels.

A cholesterol ratio of under 3.5 is considered ideal; a ratio *over* 4.5 puts you in the danger zone. The Framingham data show that a person with a ratio of 4.5 or higher is twice as likely to get a heart attack as someone whose ratio is 3.5 or less.

What makes one type of cholesterol good and the other bad? In fact, the cholesterol is all the same, but it comes wrapped in different lipoproteins. The molecules that are inside LDL wrappings get deposited on your artery walls, causing a buildup that could one day block the blood going to your heart—causing a heart attack.

On the other hand, cholesterol wrapped in HDLs gets swept to your liver, where it's disposed of—with no damage to your coronary arteries. In this way, HDL cholesterol actually protects your heart.

Daily aerobic exercise can significantly raise your HDL levels by stimulating certain muscle enzymes that produce HDLs. For example, a study at Stanford University found a 15 percent rise in HDLs among overweight men after a year-long exercise program. A group of doctors trained for the Boston Marathon several years ago and recorded an average jump of 10 points in their HDL levels, from 45 to 55. And in a study at the Institute for Aerobics Research of over 100 previously sedentary women walking at different speeds, all groups showed a 6 percent average jump in HDL levels after six months of daily walking. This was true whether they walked very quickly, or strolled at a leisurely 20-minutes-per-mile pace.

There are other ways to raise your HDL levels, too:

- If you lose weight by reducing body fat, you'll raise your HDL levels, whether or not you do any exercise.
- If you are a cigarette smoker and you quit, you'll probably boost your HDL levels five points or so. (By the way, even the *children* of smokers have been shown to have lower-than-normal HDL levels.)

- Have a drink or two of alcohol a day. This has been shown to cause a modest boost in HDL levels. Drink more than this, though, and your cholesterol profile will start to get worse instead of better.

This book has one main goal: to show that staying fit and healthy doesn't have to be complicated or confusing. In fact, a healthy life-style can be summed up by a few simple rules:

- Try to put in a half-hour or more of aerobic activity as many days each week as you can.
- Avoid smoking.
- Work hard at reducing the fatty foods you eat—especially those containing saturated fats and hydrogenated fats.
- Keep an eye on your cholesterol ratio (total cholesterol divided by HDL cholesterol), aiming for a ratio of 3.5 or less.
- If you have the time and the motivation, do a short strength workout twice a week.
- Add specific stretching and strengthening exercises to treat any "weak links" such as tight muscles or an ache-prone back.

If all of you 35 and over males follow these basic guidelines as John Jones did, you'll find yourself paying much less attention to the health-fitness hype that's flooding the media these days. There's nothing mystifying about good health: It comes from knowing what your body needs, and taking care of those needs one day at a time.

Good luck, and happy trails!

APPENDIX A

HOW EXERCISE CHANGES YOUR BODY OVER TIME

AFTER ONE WEEK

FITNESS: Although too small to notice at this point, your fitness will start improving after just a few workouts. Already, your heart muscle is getting stronger, pumping more blood with each stroke, and your leg, trunk, and arm muscles are being stimulated to produce more enzymes, triggering the growth of additional mitochondria—tiny cellular factories that convert oxygen into energy.

Expect about a 1 percent boost in your endurance after the first week, along with a drop of about one beat per minute in your resting heart rate.

BODY COMPOSITION: If you were overweight when you began your program, you may also see an early weight loss of 2 to 3 pounds. Your new program will quickly start raising levels of fat-burning enzymes in your muscles, allowing your body to burn fat more effectively.

AFTER ONE MONTH

FITNESS: By this time you'll notice a clear improvement in your endurance and your energy level. Expect about a 4 percent increase in your aerobic capacity, and a drop of about four beats per minute in your resting heart rate. You'll also be recovering faster after working out.

BODY COMPOSITION: Overweight exercisers typically lose 6 to 10 pounds after a month of exercise, especially if they cut back their normal diet by a couple of hundred calories per day.

Aerobic muscle fibers also get slightly larger by one month and show improved tone. New capillaries (tiny blood vessels) are busily growing in your working muscles, as well—an improvement that will continue steadily as long as you keep exercising.

BLOOD PRESSURE: If your blood pressure reading was higher than normal when you began your program, one month later you should expect a drop of five to seven points in your systolic pressure (the top number) and a lowering of a point or two in your diastolic pressure (the bottom number).

AFTER THREE MONTHS

FITNESS: You're now at the point of peak improvement in fitness, continuing to add about 1 percent each week to your aerobic abilities. That means you've now increased your oxygen-burning capabilities by 10 to 15 percent. Your resting heart rate will have dropped five to seven beats, on average.

BODY COMPOSITION: Your muscles may get a bit larger and more toned between one and three months, but from here on you'll need to lift weights to see any significant changes in muscle mass. Fat levels will continue to decline steadily, however. Typical weight loss for the first three months (assuming slight caloric restriction) is 12 to 17 pounds.

CHOLESTEROL: Three months is usually when the heart-protecting benefits of exercise start to show. Regular exercisers may show slight reductions in their total cholesterol levels, but the big plus about exercise is that it raises levels of protective HDL cholesterol. After three months, exercisers typically show an HDL rise of three to five percent—a small but significant increase.

BLOOD PRESSURE: Expect a 5 to 7 percent drop in systolic pressure, and a few points drop in diastolic pressure.

PSYCHOLOGICAL BENEFITS: By three months, many exercisers report increased feelings of well-being and high self-esteem and fewer feelings of sadness or anxiety.

AFTER SIX MONTHS

FITNESS: Expect a 15 to 20 percent improvement in your aerobic capacity, and a resting heart rate 10 to 15 beats per minute lower than when you started.

BODY COMPOSITION: If you began this program overweight you can expect to lose 20 to 35 pounds of body fat after six months.

CHOLESTEROL: Expect a 10 to 12 percent jump in HDL cholesterol levels after six months—significantly lowering your risk of getting heart disease or a heart attack.

BLOOD PRESSURE: Expect a reduction of 10 to 15 percent in systolic pressure, and 8 to 12 percent in diastolic pressure.

AFTER ONE YEAR

FITNESS: Gains in endurance increase slightly between six months and a year, for a 25 to 30 percent total improvement. From here on, significant gains can be made only by changing your program, and making your workouts either harder, longer, or more frequent.

BODY COMPOSITION: Your rate of fat loss will also level off between 6 and 12 months. Expect an additional 5- to 10-pound weight loss in this period.

CHOLESTEROL: HDL levels will continue to climb, though not as fast. Look for an increase of 12 to 15 percent after one year.

BLOOD PRESSURE: Expect a drop of 15 to 18 percent in your systolic pressure and 12 to 14 percent in your diastolic pressure.

APPENDIX B

MUSCLES USED IN VARIOUS AEROBIC ACTIVITIES

Front View

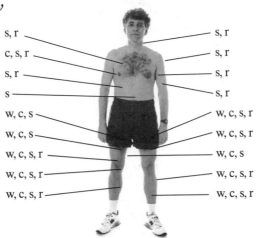

S, r	S, r
C, S, r	S, r
S, r	S, r
S	S, r
W, C, S	W, C, S, r
W, C, S	W, C, S, r
W, C, S, r	W, C, S
W, C, S, r	W, C, S, r
W, C, S, r	W, C, S, r

Rear View

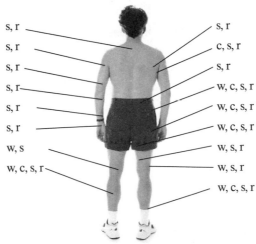

S, r	S, r
S, r	C, S, r
S, r	S, r
S, r	W, C, S, r
S, r	W, C, S, r
S, r	W, C, S, r
W, S	W, S, r
W, C, S, r	W, S, r
	W, C, S, r

W = Walking; C = Cyling; S = Swimming; R = Racket sports.

APPENDIX C

RECOMMENDED DAILY FOOD SERVINGS (U.S. DEPARTMENT OF AGRICULTURE)

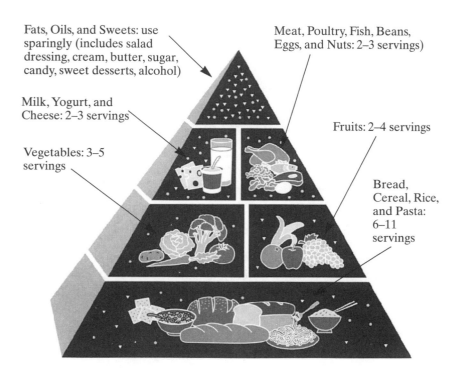

Fats, Oils, and Sweets: use sparingly (includes salad dressing, cream, butter, sugar, candy, sweet desserts, alcohol)

Meat, Poultry, Fish, Beans, Eggs, and Nuts: 2–3 servings)

Milk, Yogurt, and Cheese: 2–3 servings

Fruits: 2–4 servings

Vegetables: 3–5 servings

Bread, Cereal, Rice, and Pasta: 6–11 servings

WHAT COUNTS AS ONE SERVING?

Breads, Cereal, Rice, and Pasta
    1 slice bread
    ½ cup cooked rice or pasta
    ½ cup cooked cereal
    1 ounce ready-to-eat cereal

Vegetables
    ½ cup chopped vegetables (cooked or raw)
    1 cup leafy raw vegetables

Fruits
    1 piece raw fruit
    1 wedge melon
    ¾ cup fruit juice
    ½ cup canned fruit
    ¼ cup dried fruit

Milk, Yogurt, and Cheese
    1 cup milk or yogurt
    1 ½ to 2 ounces cheese

Meat, Poultry, Fish, Beans, Eggs, and Nuts
    2 ½ to 3 ounces cooked lean meat, poultry, or fish
    1 ½ cup cooked beans
    3 eggs
    6 tablespoons peanut butter

APPENDIX D

	% FAT	RATIO OF SATURATED FAT VS. UNSATURATED FAT
ANIMAL		
Butter	80	55 / 35
Beef	16–42	50 / 50
Lamb	19–29	60 / 40
Pork	32	45 / 55
Ham	23	45 / 55
Chicken	10–17	30 / 70
Veal	10	50 / 50
VEGETABLE		
Corn Oil	100	7 / 78
Olive Oil	100	15 / 85
Canola Oil	100	9 / 91
Margarine	81	26 / 66
Peanut Butter	50	25 / 75
Potato Chips	35	25 / 75
Cashew Nuts	48	18 / 82

APPENDIX E

Maintain routine organ functions (heart, kidneys, liver, etc.)	60–75 percent
Digesting food	10 percent
Muscular activity	15–30 percent

Most of your calories are used simply to maintain bodily functions. Your muscles are the only "discretionary" item in your daily calorie budget. This means exercise is the *only* effective way to increase the number of calories you burn each day.

APPENDIX F

Big guys take heart—the heavier you are, the more calories you burn moving around. A 165-pound man burns 6 calories per minute walking (or 360 calories an hour). That's pretty good. But a 220-pounder spins off 8 calories for every minute of walking, or 480 calories per hour. Your bulk is working in your favor each time you excercise!

CALORIES BURNED PER MINUTE	(WT.) 140 LBS.	165 LBS.	190 LBS.	220 LBS.
Walking (steady pace)	5	6	7	8
Cycling (10 mph)	6.5	7.5	8.5	10
Swimming (slow freestyle)	8	9.5	11	12.5
Raking leaves	3.5	4	4.5	5.5
Mowing the lawn	7	8.5	9.5	11
Cross-country skiing	7.5	9	10	11.5
Running (8 min. per mile)	13.5	15.5	17.5	20
Racketball	12	13.5	15	17.5
Basketball	9	10.5	12	14
Ballroom dancing	3.5	4	4.5	5

APPENDIX G

Doctors now agree that men should strive to maintain a level of body fat no higher than 20 percent of their total body mass. For women (who naturally have a higher body fat content) the cutoff point is 30 percent. Higher fat levels are associated with greater risk of heart disease, especially if the fat is mainly in your abdomen and back (the "apple" pattern), as opposed to your thighs and buttocks (the "pear" pattern).

You can have your own body fat content measured with a special pair of calipers (many physical therapists and exercise clinics have them), by being weighed underwater (a complicated process that can only be done in an exercise lab), or a technique called bioelectric impedance, in which a low electric current is passed through your body (the amount of resistance shows how much fat you have).

These methods are all complex, time-consuming, and sometimes inaccurate. A much simpler method is to develop your own relative measurement system. Using your thumb and forefinger, grab a large fold of flesh on the side of your abdomen and squeeze it, pinching the flesh between your fingers. As a general rule, if you pinch more than an inch, you're probably over your ideal fat content. The point isn't where you are now, however, but where you're going to. Measure the thickness of the skinfold, then repeat the process on the back of your upper arm.

Do this process every few weeks, recording the measurements. You should see a small but steady downward trend.

APPENDIX H

Studies have shown that if you want to know how hard you're exercising, rating your own "perceived exertion" is just as effective as complicated lab testing. The method is simple. Study the accompanying chart carefully. Then, while you're exercising, select the point on the chart that corresponds most closely to the way you feel.

Your aerobic workouts should generally be in the range of 11 through 13 on the scale. When you're lifting weights to build strength, the effort should feel harder—in the range of 15 to 17, according to your own perception.

HOW HARD DOES YOUR WORKOUT FEEL?
(THE BORG SCALE OF "PERCEIVED EXERTION")

6	
7	Very, very light
8	
9	Very light
10	
11	Fairly light
12	
13	Somewhat hard
14	
15	Hard
16	
17	Very hard
18	
19	Very, very hard
20	

APPENDIX I

As you become a more accomplished swimmer, you may want to hone your stroke a little more. The best swimmers have an edge—literally—because they've learned how to knife through water with the least possible resistance.

Here are some tips on developing an edge of your own, suggested by Columbia University swimming coach Jim Bolster:

1. Your body position in the water is all-important. When you're swimming freestyle, don't bury your head down in the water. Instead, try to hold your head up slightly so that the waterline hits the bridge of your nose. This will let your body ride on top of the water, cutting down on drag.

2. Swimming freestyle, learn to breathe comfortably on either side of your body. This way you can take a breath every three strokes, instead of every two, helping you to swim in a straight line and developing your muscles in a more balanced way.

3. Concentrate on feeling the water during each arm pull. You should feel your cupped hand "catch" the water as soon as it hits the surface. Focus then on using your arm's full length, from your fingertips to your underarm, to push the water down and under you.

4. Whatever stroke you use, get a good push off the wall each time you make a turn at the end of a lap. This is when you're moving your fastest, so use your momentum to glide at least one full body length before resuming your stroke.

APPENDIX J

DETERMINING YOUR AEROBIC LIMIT

Your aerobic limit is the hardest effort you can do without switching over to emergency anaerobic energy supplies in your muscles. If you want to improve your cardiovascular fitness, the idea is to work as closely to this limit as you can, without going over it.

Scientists have found that this aerobic limit occurs when your heart is beating at about 75% of its maximum rate. (Maximum heart rate, measured in beats per minute, is approximately equal to 220 minus your age.)

If you stop briefly to measure your heart rate during a workout, you'll be able to tell how hard you're working. If you're below or even with your aerobic limit, you're building health and endurance. If your heart rate is more than ten beats *over* this limit, however, you're no longer working aerobically—and it's time to ease up on the pace.

AGE	MAXIMUM HEART RATE (beats per minute)	AEROBIC LIMIT (beats per minute)
35	185	139
40	180	135
45	175	132
50	170	128
55	165	124
60	160	120
65	155	117
70	150	113

Aerobic Fitness

Walking, by Casey Meyers. New York: Random House, 1992, $12.00. To order: 800-726-0600.

Effective Cycling, by John Forester. Cambridge, MA: MIT Press, 1988, $17.50. To order: 617-625-8569.

Swimming for Total Fitness, by Jane Katz, EdD. New York: Doubleday, 1993, $17.50. To order: 800-323-9872. (To order the Jane Katz pool calisthenics video, *Water Exercises Techniques Workout,* call 800-967-5469.)

Healthy Heart

Dr. Dean Ornish's Program for Reversing Heart Disease, by Dean Ornish, MD. New York: Random House, 1992, $15.00. To order: 800-726-0600.

Weight Control

Living Without Dieting, by John Foreyt, PhD, and G. Ken Goodrick, PhD. New York: Warner Books, 1992, $10.99. To Order: 212-522-7200

Back Care

Back Care Basics, by Mary Pullig Schatz, MD. Berkeley, CA: Rodmell Press, 1992, $19.95. To order: 510-841-3123.

Treat Your Own Back, by Robin McKenzie. Waikanae, New Zealand: Spinal Publications Ltd., 1985, $10.00. To order: 800-367-7393.

The BackPower Program, by David Imrie, MD, and Lu Barbuto, DC. New York: John Wiley and Sons, 1990, $12.95. To order: 800-225-5945.

Healing Back Pain, by John Sarno, MD. New York: Warner Books, 1991, $9.99. To order: 212-522-7200.

Strength Training

Be Strong, by Wayne Westcott, PhD. Dubuque, IA: William C. Brown, 1993, $12.00. To order: 800-338-5578.

Fitness Weight Training, by Tom Baechle and Roger Earle. Champaign, IL: Human Kinetics, 1995, $14.95. To order: 800-747-4457.

Stretching and Yoga

Stretching, by Bob Anderson. Bolinas, CA: Shelter Publications, 1980, $12.00. To order: 415-868-0280.

The American Yoga Association Beginner's Manual, by Alice Christensen. New York: Simon and Schuster, 1987, $15.00. To order: 800-223-2348.

The Sivananda Companion to Yoga, by Lucy Lidell. New York: Simon and Schuster, 1983, $14.00. To order: 800-223-2348.

Stress Reduction

The Relaxation Response, by Herbert Benson, MD. New York: Avon Books, 1976, $5.99. To order: 800-238-0658.

Creative Stress Management, by Jonathan Smith, PhD. Englewood Cliffs, NJ: Prentice Hall, 1992, $23.00. To order: 800-922-0579.

General Reference

Exercise Physiology, by William McArdle, Frank Katch, and Victor Katch. Baltimore, MD: Williams & Wilkins, 1991, $57.95. To order: 800-638-0672.

INDEX